ORGAN TRANSPLANTS
AND ETHICS

Organ Transplants and Ethics

DAVID LAMB

Avebury

Aldershot • Brookfield USA • Hong Kong • Singapore • Sydney

Published by
Avebury
Ashgate Publishing Limited
Gower House
Croft Road
Aldershot
Hants GU11 3HR
England

Ashgate Publishing Company
Old Post Road
Brookfield
Vermont 05036
USA

First published by Routledge in 1990
Reprinted 1996 by Avebury

British Library Cataloguing in Publication Data
Lamb, David, 1942-
    Organ transplants and ethics. - (Avebury series in
    philosophy)
    1.Transplantation of organs, tissues, etc. - Moral and
    ethical aspects.
    I.Title
    174.2'5

Library of Congress Cataloging-in-Publication Data
Library of Congress Catalog Card Number: 96-85558

ISBN 1 85972 507 4

Printed in Great Britain by
Antony Rowe Ltd, Chippenham, Wiltshire

FOR
STORM

CONTENTS

ACKNOWLEDGEMENTS

This book arose in response to an invitation to participate in a debate on the ethics of organ transplantation which took place in January 1987 in the Medical School of the University of Manchester. I am grateful to the organizers of that meeting and members of the audience for directing my attention to many ethical problems in this area. I have also benefited considerably from discussions and correspondence with Dr Anna Maria Bernasconi, a member of the Italian Parliament with a specific interest in ethics and legislation on organ transplantation. I wish to thank the President of the Committee on Social Affairs in the Camera Dei Deputati, Rome, for the opportunity to air some of the topics discussed in Chapters 2 and 3 of this book in a public debate.

A short version of the chapter dealing with proposals to procure transplantable organs from anencephalic infants was presented to a conference on Health, Economics, Law, and Medicine, at the University of Aberdeen in the Summer of 1989. I would like to thank members of the Philosophy Department at Aberdeen for their hospitality. I am also grateful for encouragement from Professor R.J. Butler and the Tonbridge Philosophical Society.

During later stages of preparation many valuable criticisms were made by Susan Easton, Heather Draper, and Cindy Pateras, who are not in any way responsible for any errors that may remain. I am deeply indebted to numerous writers whose work I have referred to throughout the text. Thanks also to Lynn Evans for secretarial assistance throughout the whole project, and to Richard Stoneman of Routledge for his encouragement and support. Finally I would like to thank Kate Morrall, also of Routledge, for her efforts during the final stages of preparation.

David Lamb
Department of Philosophy, University of Manchester

INTRODUCTION

Moral and philosophical issues have been raised in relation to every aspect of organ transplantation. These include the morality of excising organs from a healthy donor, and related problems regarding an individual's consent to have organs removed for the benefit of others. These problems are not restricted to live donation: cadaveric organ procurement raises problems regarding the definition of and criteria for death, and raises further questions of fundamental moral concern over the authorization of organ removal. Both secular and religious belief systems throughout the world stress moral affinities between respect for living beings and cadavers. The time may be approaching when every part of a cadaver can be utilized for the benefit of organ recipients and experimental research. It is necessary, therefore, to ask whether there is a moral limit to what can be done to a dead body. Should appeals to the sanctity of the human body outweigh the interests of those who have an urgent need for bodily parts? These problems are, so far, unresolved. So too are the problems bound up with the procurement of organs and their allocation. Technical skills in transplant surgery have rapidly outpaced society's ability, or willingness, to supply adequate resources. When formulating ethical guidelines in this area it is therefore necessary to consider competing moral standpoints: should utilitarian or egalitarian principles underpin social policy options for the procurement and allocation of transplantable organs? Does a person who needs an organ in order to live have a moral claim to the organs of another being? There does not appear to be any firm consensus with regard to this question. For some the interests of the living outweigh those of the dead and consequently they see nothing unethical in the routine harvesting of cadaveric organs. Another standpoint expresses concern that such practices would, in some

1

way, imperil individual autonomy and undermine the basis of altruism. Opinions also vary with regard to the removal of organs from beings who are deemed to be incapable of benefiting from them, such as aborted foetuses, dying anencephalic infants, and patients in persistent vegetative states. Other ethical problems raised by organ transplantation are the fair distribution of organs to those awaiting transplants, whether the human body is a marketable commodity, the physician's obligations to both donor and recipient, and problems arising out of the fact that organ transplantation introduces the problem of a third party – the donor – between doctor and patient.

These issues draw attention to one of the most profound problems concerning the degree of one individual's moral obligation to another. To what extent is an individual responsible for the provision of well-being for others? This question – 'Am I my brother's keeper?' – predates modern transplant surgery, and is raised whenever serious ethical issues are considered. In the context of the problems addressed in this book the obligations of one individual to another are measured, not merely by the extent of donations of money or possessions, but by the donation of parts of an individual which are excised and secured in the body of another.

It is inescapable that a book which investigates the ethical issues of organ transplants will be concerned with practical matters, and will draw heavily from the kind of medical sources which are said to fall outside the parameters of philosophical enquiry. The objection might be made that the approach taken in this book, as with my earlier book, *Death, Brain Death and Ethics* (Lamb, 1985), focuses primarily on empirical issues at the expense of the purely philosophical. But this objection misses the point of the practical philosophy outlined here, which is based on the belief that conceptual issues should be examined in their practical context. Such questions as whether or not to ventilate a patient, and whether or not it is appropriate to excise transplantable organs, are practical problems facing the physician, the patient and relatives, which cannot be neatly separated from broader ethical, philosophical and ontological matters. Underpinning therapy decisions in the context of organ transplantation are the deeper questions concerning what it means to be a human being and what obligations humans should have towards others. Guiding decisions in these areas is a mass of empirical knowledge, scientific

2

theory and philosophical beliefs concerning what it means to say that someone is dead or alive, or that their prognosis is hopeless, or that they are competent to make a decision, or that other considerations should override a competent decision, and the very meaning of therapeutic intervention itself.

The problems raised in relation to organ transplantation are not the kind that are easily resolved by reference to the respective merits of neo-Aristotelian, neo-Kantian, or any variety of utilitarianism, or any other philosophical school. A distinction between applied and practical philosophy may be appropriate here. Many exponents of applied philosophy appear to believe that one must first determine the respective merits of the competing theories of, for example, Aristotle, Kant and Bentham, and then apply a methodology attributed to the winner to the problem under consideration. To the exponent of practical philosophy there is something artificial about the application of a philosophical system like sticking plaster to problems in medicine, law, education, science, or business. It is far from clear that philosophy, applied in this way, is capable of solving anything. Although some of the ethical dilemmas associated with organ transplants could well be resolved by means of attention to the background principles, other dilemmas may be resolved by advances in technology, developments in medical knowledge, or even a shift in societal attitudes towards the allocation of certain resources. Thus advances in immunosuppressive therapy, which eliminate a need for a close genetic match between donor and recipient, can resolve ethical dilemmas faced by relatives under pressure to donate organs. Advances in pre-natal screening techniques may resolve problems bound up with the procurement of organs from dying neonates, but they may simply shift the problem to a stage early in pregnancy when a decision whether or not to abort is required.

The opening chapter of this book summarizes the history of organ transplantation in order to emphasize its twin aspects: high-risk experiment and routine therapy. Ethical problems are therefore located, and sometimes resolved, in the dialectic between experimental research and clinical routine. This distinction is important, for it draws attention to two different classes of ethical problems. In the first case it is appropriate to question whether hopelessly incurable individuals should be subjected to experimental methods when benefit is more likely to accrue to others as a result of perfection in technique. It should be stressed in this context that just as the techniques of transplant surgery were experimental in the early stages, so too were the ethics. Organ transplantation, like many other developments in a scientific age, did not begin with access to a fully articulated system of ethical rules to guide researchers. These rules evolved, so to speak, along with the techniques. In the second case, where organ transplantation is routine therapy, the appropriate ethical questions are bound up with the availability of procedures and the equitable distribution of resources.

Cadaveric organ transplants highlight the fact that one person's death can offer the hope of life for others, but it forces discussion of the mechanism of death and emphasizes a need for a publicly acceptable definition of death with reliable criteria and tests. Recent inquiries into this problem form the basis of the second and third chapters. Part of the problem is that organs removed from dead persons must, if they are to be successfully transplanted, still retain some life in them – and it is therefore apparent that the body of the donor still has some life in it. For many people this raises problems about the determination of death in cases involving organ donation. This issue is one of the most fundamental in the ethical controversies associated with organ transplantations, and it continues to generate confusion and moral uncertainty. Chapter 2 examines the development of brain-related criteria for death and assesses the philosophical status of the brainstem concept of death which is employed in the UK and several other countries. Chapter 3 examines more recent, and highly controversial, proposals to expand the boundaries of brain death so as to include as potential cadaveric organ donors patients in various non-cognitive states who, according to existing moral and legal guidelines, are deemed to be alive. The underlying theme, in both Chapters 2 and 3, is a moral imperative to strive for and maintain a precise formulation of a concept of death which yields unambiguous clinical criteria.

The establishment of precise guidelines concerning the determination of death is bound up with suspension of therapy and removal of transplantable organs if required. But a proposed definition of death must be separated from proposals for euthanasia and utilitarian requirements for more transplantable organs. The author's opposition to euthanasia (either passive or active, voluntary or non-voluntary) was expressed in *Down the Slippery Slope* (Lamb, 1988) and is maintained here. Nevertheless, there are many people who see in discussions about transplant procedures a need to repeat their opinions in favour of accelerated death. When the body's mechanism fails, it is often asked, just how many parts should be supplied in order to keep it going? Is there not a point at which we should call for a halt to the therapy and either allow or assist death to bring down the final curtain? These questions have an argument in favour of euthanasia built into them. This book cannot answer them directly, any more than it can state how much life is enough. But the case for euthanasia is being put forward strongly and repeatedly by intellectuals and the media. I have a suspicion that behind the widespread endorsement of euthanasia in the media, and the volumes of philosophical books endorsing one or more categories of euthanasia, lies a vague and implicit awareness that the benefits of recent biomedical advances cannot be universally distributed without a fundamental re-distribution of resources. Support for euthanasia reflects the interests of a class, social group or nation, whose material interests may suffer if medicine's ability to effect a dramatic reduction in mortality rates were applied on a large scale to the poor and ethnic unwanted. Far better, it would seem, if widespread belief in the value of euthanasia were encouraged. The 90 per cent of Dutch economics undergraduates who in a recent opinion poll expressed support for 'compulsory euthanasia on unspecified groups of people to streamline the economy' (Fenigsen, 1989:25) may well have explicitly expressed beliefs which are implicitly maintained by those who call for the imposition of limits on organ transplantation.

This book does not offer any solution to the problem of how to provide the maximum benefits of medicine, in particular organ transplantation. But it does express the view that, whatever benefits transplantation can provide, the procurement and allocation of organs should proceed according to principles of equity together with policies which maintain respect for the human body. To this end Chapter 4 examines ethical problems raised by proposals to procure foetal tissue for transplantation purposes. Chapter 5 examines the problems inherent in recent proposals to procure organs from dying neonates, whilst Chapter 6 examines the problems of cadaveric organ procurement as well as policies for obtaining replacement organs and tissues from living humans and various non-human sources. The final chapter assesses policy options for the procurement and allocation of organs, some of which are under consideration for adoption in the form of legal directives in several countries.

Although several philosophers and lawyers have contributed to discussions of biomedical issues in the UK, there is an appalling absence of informed Parliamentary discussion. Like the periodic debates on the restoration of capital punishment, euthanasia bills are occasionally introduced and from time to time proposals to amend the Abortion Act are put forward. Otherwise, legislation on bioethical issues proceeds in a rather *ad hoc* manner, as in the case of the recently introduced bill outlawing the sale of organs. There is clearly a need for a standing commission on issues related to contemporary bioethical problems, akin to the President's Commission which functioned for over a decade in the USA. It is hoped that this book, for all its imperfections, will stimulate demand for such a commission, whose brief will be to monitor existing legislation on organ procurement and distribution in the light of developments in surgical technique and scientific possibility.

1

TRANSPLANTS: EXPERIMENT OR THERAPY?

And the Lord God caused the man to fall into a deep sleep;
and while he was sleeping, he took one of the man's ribs
and closed up the place with flesh ... and made a woman
from the rib he had taken out of the man.

(Genesis 2:21,22)

The idea of organ and tissue transplantation goes back to earliest
records. According to the book of Genesis, Eve, the first woman,
was fashioned out of a rib harvested from Adam, the first donor.
The idea of taking bone, skin, or organs from one person and
transplanting them into another has been a subject of fascination
and intrigue since earliest times. Yet until the twentieth century
the dream of creating a healthy whole person by transplantation
remained in the realm of mythology and the miraculous. Early
attempts at blood transfusion met with no success until knowledge
of different blood types and their mutual compatibility or incom-
patibility was discovered. This meant that many attempts at blood
transfusion during the eighteenth century resulted in charges of
homicide before several European courts outlawed the practice.
However, blood transfusion was widely used in the 1914–18 War
when blood banks were created to store blood. This, perhaps, was
one of the most important features in the early stages of the
history of transplantation.

But blood is self-replaceable, and although there have been
considerable ethical discussions about the policies for collection
and distribution of blood, they do not address the kind of ethical
and philosophical problems associated with the transplantation
of non-regenerating solid organs, such as kidneys, hearts, lungs,
pancreases, and livers.

Transplantation of non-vital organs has steadily increased during

7

the twentieth century. Skin grafts began in the late 1920s. This procedure is usually applied as a temporary measure in cases of burns. Recent experiments with cultured skin, however, suggest that procurement from donors may one day be unnecessary. Under appropriate conditions skin can be stored and there are now skin and bone banks, where bone is stored for treatment of the skeletal system.

Corneal transplants actually began in 1905, although the operation did not become routine until the 1940s. In 1983 a corneal transplant service was set up in the UK to encourage corneal donation. Improvements in storage techniques now allow corneas to be stored for up to thirty days. The Corneal Tissue Act of 1986 greatly enhanced cadaveric procurement in the UK by allowing non-medical personnel to remove corneas. Since 1944, when the world's first eye-bank was opened in the Manhattan Eye, Ear, and Throat Hospital, eye banks have become an integral part of most countries' health-care systems. In recent years more than 95 per cent of corneal transplant recipients have had their sight restored. In 1986 over 28,000 corneal transplants were performed in the USA. Current research indicates that retinal transplants may soon be possible for many people who go blind in later life. Professor John Marshall, at the Institute of Opthalmology in London, has been studying ways of renewing cells of the retina as they wear out. It is hoped that by removing the pigment epithelium cells from a healthy part of the eye, then growing them in a laboratory, before transplanting them to the diseased part of the eye, patients suffering from age-related macular degeneration (and possibly patients with the inherited disease of the retina known as retinitis pigmentosa) may be able to benefit (Anon., *New Scientist*, 1989:25).

The modern transplant era, however, began with the transplantation of non-regenerating vital organs in the 1950s, but its antecedents can be traced back to the turn of the century when Dr Alexis Carrel and Dr Charles C. Guthrie developed the technique of suturing blood vessels. Then, in 1902, an Austrian surgeon, Dr Emmerick Ullman, removed a kidney from a dog and kept it functioning in the body of another dog for a few days. The eventual failure of this transplant revealed the problem of rejection, and it was discovered in further experiments that successful transplants depend on a close genetic resemblance between donor and recipient.

There are four distinct types of transplant which are significant for the assessment of potential rejection. First, there are *autografts*, which are transplants of an organ or tissue within the same individual, such as skin or bone marrow, from one part of the body to another. Second, there are *homografts*, from one individual to another within the same species. Third, there are *heterografts*, between individuals of different species, usually animals to humans, which are also known as *xenografts*. Fourth, there are *isografts*, between genetically identical individuals, such as identical twins.

The major breakthrough in understanding rejection had to wait until Dr Peter Medawar, winner of the 1960 Nobel Prize, explained how the body's immunization system recognizes foreign bodies that enter it by means of markers or *antigens*, and then rejects foreign matter by means of the production of *antibodies*. This knowledge led to the development of tissue-typing, where the donor's and recipient's tissues are examined with a view to compatibility, such that the antigens of both tissues are sufficiently similar to prevent recognition as alien bodies and thus avoid exciting the destructive immune system response. In recent years great efforts have been made to overcome the rejection problem, without which surgical technique would be insufficient. Throughout the 1960s and 1970s drugs were developed which lessened the organism's ability to develop antibodies. But many of these had the unfortunate effect of weakening the recipient's immune system. However, a major breakthrough occurred in 1983 when a Swiss pharmaceutical company produced cyclosporin which selectively inhibits the rejection of foreign tissues without damaging their ability to combat viruses and bacteria. The ability to control tissue rejection marks the transition from the era of transplantation as an experimental therapy to the era of organ transplantation as routine therapy.

Yet in another sense, cyclosporin introduces a further aspect of experimentation. Cyclosporin is synthesized from a soil fungus; it does not attack white blood cell production in the bone marrow, as most other immunosuppressive agents do. Its obvious benefit is that it can forestall rejection without destroying host defences. It is usually employed with other immunosuppressives and is the most widely used drug for the combat of rejection. It reduces complications, shortens hospital stay, and has extended the range of transplants, offering benefit to high risk patients, including those with high degrees of immunological reactivity. But like other immunosuppressives it has serious side-effects, which might include 'tremors, convulsions, swelling and inflammation of the gums, abnormal growth of body hair, and an increased incidence of lymphoma and Kaposi's sarcoma' (New York Task Force, 1988:20). There are also possible toxic side-effects which may affect other organs, in particular the kidneys. Improvements in combating side-effects and toxicity have been made – including means of finding the best combinations of drugs – and research is under way.

The major ethical problems concerning organ transplantation relate to the replacement of solid organs, such as kidneys, hearts, lungs, pancreases, and livers. Here the dialectic between experiment and therapy highlights the ethical problems. In the initial stages of solid organ transplants the ethical problems turned on the morality of conducting experiments on seemingly hopeless and desperate cases. But where transplantation has become routine therapy, the ethical problems are bound up with the procurement and allocation of organs, although considerable problems concerning experimentation occur as the transplant programme expands into new fields.

The first transplant of a non-regenerative vital organ was a kidney transplant performed by Dr David Hume in Boston in 1951, who used a cadaver donor in an unsuccessful attempt to save his patient's life. During the next four years Dr Hume and his colleague, Dr Joseph E. Murray, performed a further ten kidney transplants using cadaver donors, but most of their patients died shortly after the operation. However, on 11 February 1953, a renal transplant was performed on a patient who survived for six months. Then in 1954 Dr Murray and Dr John Merrill successfully carried out what is recognized as the world's first living donor transplantation between monozygotic twins. Richard Herrick, aged 22, received a kidney from his identical twin brother, Ronald, and lived for a further eight years with good renal function before dying of a heart attack (Varga, 1984:214).

Following successes with identical twins later transplants were conducted with fraternal twins and close relatives, although the techniques were highly experimental. In 1959 a kidney transplant between fraternal twins was achieved as a result of 'using total body irradiation in sublethal dose to breach a modest immunological barrier' (Lyons, 1970:40). Because of rejection problems the

10

early kidney transplants from live donors were generally restricted to twins or close relatives, thus introducing a new dimension of moral pressure on the relatives of victims of kidney disease.

During the next twenty years skill in antigen matching and advances in immunosuppressive therapy transformed the renal transplant programme. By the mid 1980s transplant surgeons were achieving success rates of over 80 per cent survival for at least five years among those receiving kidneys from live related donors. The first successful cadaveric renal transplant was in 1962. At that time the rejection rate from cadaveric donors was high, but by the mid 1980s the success rate had risen dramatically to around 60 per cent five-year survival, with an average of 8.2 years before rejection. The annual rate of kidney transplants continues to increase. In 1985 7,452 renal transplants were performed in Europe and in 1986, 8,976 kidneys were transplanted in the USA. The number world-wide was 21,000.

The best results are obtained with good histocompatibility and antigen matching. The best match is between identical twins, where the average survival is 29.2 years, followed by non-identical siblings and parents, with a 12.1-year average before rejection.

Not only do kidney transplants provide a better quality of life than dialysis, the cost of transplants is comparatively less expensive than alternative therapy. In the USA in 1983 dialysis cost an individual an estimated $35,000 each year, whereas post-surgery treatment following transplantation was between $5,000 and $8,000, with a better quality of life. In the UK, according to the Director of the UK Transplant Service at Bristol, a kidney transplant lasting five years would save the NHS £60,000 at 1982 prices (Bradley, 1988:1377). As a general rule the cost of a successful transplant plus one year of post-operative therapy amounts to less than the cost of one year of the cheapest form of chronic dialysis. After the first year the costs are negligible (Report of the Conference of European Health Ministers, 1987).

There are, however, many residual problems with renal transplants. Many patients reject their grafts and have to return to dialysis, or receive another graft. In the USA 1,500 return to dialysis each year. Complications can occur. Approximately 80 per cent of kidney recipients develop infection at some time after their transplant, and of these for 25 per cent the infection leads to death. The most serious infections involve the lungs. Then there are the risks of side-effects of the immunosuppressive drugs, which include hypertension, hepatitis, and cancer (New York Task Force, 1988:14; also Toledo-Pereyra, 1987; Vincenti, Parfrey, and Briggs, 1986).

Nevertheless, a successful renal transplant is preferable to any alternative therapy. It offers respite from continuous dependence on dialysis machines. It provides a better quality of life for less expense than dialysis. Patients have returned to full normal health after a kidney graft; and even more, as displayed at the Transplant Olympics in September 1987 at Innsbruck. And one successful kidney recipient among the 400 or so transplant recipients in the World Transplant Games in Singapore, 1989, has achieved times of 54.6 seconds for the 400 metres and 11.68 seconds for the 100 metres since his transplant (the *Guardian*, 29 May 1989). Moreover, results are improving each year as better methods of postoperative therapy are developed.

The full ethical and broader philosophical implications of the transplant era dawned on 3 December 1967, in Cape Town, when Louis Washinsky received the first heart transplant from surgeon Dr Christian Barnard. Washinsky lived only for a further 18 days. Barnard's second patient, Philip Blaiberg, was to survive for 84 weeks.

The moral debate which followed is by no means resolved, but one conclusion can be drawn: that operation on Washinsky ended all beliefs that medicine was a value-free science. Organ transplantation could no longer be regarded just as a scientific possibility, but as a fundamental issue concerning human relationships. The removal of a healthy organ from a donor had to be seen as a moral as well as a medical issue. The issues raised by the first cardiac transplant not only covered the extent to which it was considered acceptable to strive in order to maintain life; problems were raised concerning the very nature and value of human life, and the numerous moral problems which are raised by the tampering with human organs. Moreover, the significance of the Barnard operation revealed the extent to which, in the public mind, heart transplants were not perceived as mere replacements of a pump and machinery for circulating blood. It revealed the moral, symbolic and cultural significance of the heart.

The Barnard operation immediately initiated a world-wide spate of similar attempts. In 1968, 107 heart transplants were performed by 64 teams in 24 countries. Critics argued that the programme was too hasty, and that the competitive attitude displayed by some teams was undignified. In fact the British heart transplant era began in an atmosphere of ballyhoo in 1968, when one cardiac team was strongly criticized for posing in front of TV cameras wearing 'I'm backing Britain' flags and buttons (Sandler, 1968). That same year the *Lancet* ran a headline 'Too many too soon', with an editorial suggesting that surgical skill in heart transplants had run ahead of knowledge about the control of rejection and infection, and against the advice of immunologists and pathologists. In fact the poor performance of 21 UK heart recipients between 3 December and 7 June 1968–9 suggested that too much priority had been given far too early to heart transplants.

Similar conclusions were drawn in America. An editorial column in the *Journal of the American Medical Association* expressed the problem: 'Despite the advances made in immuno-suppressive therapy, the problem of maintaining a viable organ in a hostile environment, without fatally compromising the host's ability to resist disease, remains the central problem of transplantation' (Editorial, *JAMA*, 1968:2835). The problem was that the immunosuppressive drugs then used – azathioprine (Imuran), corticosteroids (Prednisone in particular), and antilymphocyte serum (ALS) or antilymphocyte globulin (ALG) – produced a 'sharp reduction in the ability of the body to defend itself against bacterial, viral and fungal invasion' (Moore, 1968:2490). The very efforts to combat rejection lowered the body's natural resistance to invasive substances such as bacteria and viruses. In 1969 Helen B. Taussig of the Johns Hopkins School of Medicine warned against the premature claims of cardiac transplantation: 'Some day, we will know how a person can develop tolerance to one organ and still fight off other foreign substances and infections. Until such time, cardiac transplantation will remain a research procedure' (Taussig, 1969:9). In the USA between 1967 and the mid-1970s only 162 heart transplants took place. Of these, 104 died within 3 months and 20 survived for only between 4 and 6 months. Many transplant teams disbanded.

But at the very time that cardiac transplantation was being criticized as a risky, premature and experimental course, kidney transplants were becoming routine. The success of kidney transplantation in the 1960s was due in part to the development of azathioprine and the fact that rejection of a kidney graft is not as great as for the heart. But kidneys had another advantage: if a kidney was rejected it could be removed and the patient returned to dialysis until another kidney became available. The same did not apply to cardiac transplants, where there was no option of a new machine, but simply a decision whether to let the patient succumb to the destruction of the organ through rejection or administer large doses of potentially lethal immunosuppresive drugs and possibly destroy the body's ability to combat foreign elements.

A high price was paid for the premature claims regarding cardiac transplantation. There was too much hype, immediate false hope, followed by apathy. To this day a considerable degree of public apathy towards organ donation can be attributed to the publicity, followed by poor results, during the early stages of cardiac transplantation, together with little awareness of the steady improvements achieved during the next twenty years.

Although the cardiac transplantation programme did not expand during the 1970s an American team, led by Dr Norman Shumway at Stanford University, continued, and by the late 1970s were beginning to show results that re-established the therapeutic value of cardiac transplantation. By the mid-1980s they were producing considerable improvements in survival rates. Thus in 1986 the US national one-year survival rate was 75 to 85 per cent (New York Task Force, 1988:15). With near satisfactory immunosuppressive therapy cardiac transplantation is becoming part of routine therapy and its expansion is inevitable. In the 21 countries which make up the Council of Europe, 2,456 heart transplants had been performed by January 1985 (Report of the Conference of European Health Ministers, 1987). Between 1983 and 1985 the number of US heart transplant centres increased from 12 to 71. By 1986, 1,002 hearts had been transplanted in 84 US centres, and by then Medicare had accepted cardiac transplantation as 'a medically reasonable and necessary service' for adults, when performed in hospitals which met certain criteria (New York Task Force, 1988:15). In children, however, the rejection rate is greater, and cardiac transplantation remains experimental. They are also subject to risks of side-effects from cyclosporin, such as the possibility of retarded growth, hypertension and malignant neoplasms.

Each year over 400 cardiac transplants are performed worldwide with good prospects of survival rates. Over 80 per cent survival rates for one year have been achieved. According to Mr John Dark, Director of the cardio-pulmonary unit at the Freeman

Hospital, Newcastle, in the UK, 'the survival rate for someone well enough to walk into hospital for a transplant is now 93 per cent' (the *Guardian*, 29 May 1989). The longest surviving heart recipient is a Frenchman, Emmanuel Vitria, who received a transplant in 1968 and is still believed to be alive in 1989.

It is still an expensive operation. In the USA the cost of cardiac transplantation is estimated to be between $50,000 and $150,000, which includes the first year after surgery with both hospitalization and outpatient care. In the USA it is frequently financed by insurance arrangements, although Medicare and federal funding can be made available to eligible persons (Schroeder and Hunt, 1987:3145).

Opinions regarding costs of transplant operations vary considerably. It is not easy to assess the real cost of transplant surgery in isolation from other work performed in a hospital. It is labour-intensive, which indicates expense, but much of the background research as well as side-benefits of transplant technology have potential benefits for other aspects of health care. For example, cyclosporin was developed with organ transplants in mind, but recent research suggests that it may also be effective in the early treatment of diabetes. 'If this proved true', says Franklin (1988:36), 'thousands of children might be spared insulin injections and saved from premature death due to diabetes.' Any attempt to isolate the financial aspects of particular forms of health care will inevitably depend upon drawing arbitrary boundaries, and for this reason the appeal to costs should not play an overriding role when evaluating therapy decisions concerning transplantation.

The range of patients capable of benefiting from organ transplants has extended over the past decade. Cyclosporin therapy nowadays allows consideration of patients over the age of 55 for cardiac replacement if they are otherwise vigorous. But whilst the impact of immunosuppressive therapy has dramatically enhanced cardiac transplantation, its potential side-effects are indicative of its experimental aspects. According to one survey cyclosporin 'produces nephrotoxicity in 70 to 100 per cent of patients, and it is also toxic to the liver and the central nervous system' (Kirkpatrick, 1987:2999). However, this toxic reaction is usually reversed when administration of the drug is stopped or dosage reduced (ibid:2999). Moreover, many cardiac transplant centres now employ multiple drug immunosuppressive regimens in an effort to lower doses of several drugs without overlapping toxicities.

At Stanford the regimen includes 'administration of cyclosporin, azathioprine, and low dose Prednisone on a long-term basis and the use of rabbit antithymocyte globulin (RATG) or OKT3 for resistent rejection episodes' (Schroeder and Hunt, 1987:3144). Nevertheless, long-term immunosuppressive therapy may result in an increased tendency of patients to develop lymphoproliferative malignancies. Each immunosuppressive drug has its own toxicity (ibid:3144).

Apart from improvements in immunosuppressive monitoring and treatment, the success rate in cardiac transplants, which is now matching renal transplants, is also due to improvements in criteria for selection of recipients. As a general rule the patient must have a terminal cardiac condition for which no alternative treatment is available. But developments in conventional high-risk surgery have increased the potential for alternative therapy, allowing more stringent criteria concerning patient selection for transplants. Some patients may have greater potential benefit from conventional high-risk surgery. For example, 'some patients with coronary heart disease who continue to have angina might be more suitable for angioplasty, or repeated coronary artery bypass surgery' (Schroeder and Hunt, 1987:3142). In some cases valve replacement or the implantation of an automatic defibrillator would be pursued before resorting to cardiac transplantation. Some patients have responded sufficiently well to steroid therapy to preclude the need for transplantation (ibid:3142). On the other hand improvements in prognostic skills regarding other potentially terminal conditions would count among selection factors when choosing patients for heart transplantation.

Apart from kidneys and hearts there are lung, liver, cornea, bone, bone marrow, skin, ovary, testicle, nerve, middle ear, small intestine, and pancreatic tissue transplants (with progress being made towards successful whole pancreatic transplants), and the number of organs that can be transplanted is still increasing.

Liver transplantation was pioneered by Sir Roy Calne in Cambridge, UK, and Thomas Starzl in Pittsburgh, USA. The first successful transplant was in 1963, although the patient only survived for a further 22 days (Varga, 1984:217). However, after many disappointments new immunosuppressive drugs have begun to raise success rates, such that liver transplants now have 70 per cent success and the number of operations is steadily increasing. In 1982 there were 21 in the UK, but in 1987 there were 172 (the

Guardian, 30 December 1988). In the USA, there were 12 in 1983 and 36 in 1985 (New York Task Force, 1988:5). By 1987 over 900 liver transplants had been performed in the world. Of the 568 who received them in the USA, 269 were still alive in 1987 (Kirkpatrick, 1987:2999).

Nevertheless, liver transplantation is experimental and is regarded as a high-risk therapy, provided for congenital diseases in children and for acquired diseases in adults. But before transplantation is considered the patient must have irreversible chronic progressive liver disease and all other forms of therapy must be exhausted before acceptance into a liver transplant programme. The best results have been obtained in children with biliary atresia and metabolic defects (New York Task Force, 1988:16). At present post-operative success requires constant vigilance through numerous life-threatening complications. Liver transplantation, as Sir Roy Calne says, is 'an extremely formidable operative procedure in which major physiological disturbances are necessary and a single error at any stage is likely to lead to the patient's death' (Calne, 1987:xiii). It is extremely expensive, and is probably the most costly transplant operation currently performed. One estimate in 1985 put the cost of a liver transplant at between $75,000 and $240,000, which was approximately twice the estimated cost of a heart transplant.

Nevertheless, greater skills in liver transplant surgery will inevitably focus attention upon several ethical problems concerning organ donation. In August 1989, surgeons at the Princess Alexandria Hospital, Brisbane, Australia, opened the door to liver transplants from living donors when they removed half a liver from a 29-year-old mother, cut it down in size and transplanted it into her 1-year-old son (Anderson, 1989:26). According to reliable predictions, the remaining half of the mother's liver should grow back to its normal size within ten weeks whilst the infant's liver will grow with the child. The technique of cutting down livers has developed over a number of years through the use of adult cadaver donors whose livers are too large for transplantation into infants. If living liver donation becomes routine then this procedure could save the lives of many children who are dying because of a shortage of cadaver donors. At present, proposals are confined to transplantation from parents and siblings, although it is possible for non-relatives to become donors. This, however,

17

raises both legal and ethical questions concerning the possibility of people offering to sell part of their liver.

Transplantation of the pancreas may involve the whole pancreas or segments. It is usually performed on patients with insulin diabetes mellitus. The first clinical pancreas transplant was performed by surgeons at the University of Minnesota in 1966, but the operation is very infrequent, and highly experimental. Despite a high incidence of surgical complications and patient mortality there has been a slight increase in the number of pancreatic transplants. Between 1978 and 1985, the world-wide number of pancreatic transplants was 713; but during 1985, 214 transplants were performed in centres throughout the world.

Allogenic bone marrow transplants are increasingly performed on persons who are unable to produce the white blood cells necessary for destroying·infectious bacteria, and long-term survival is common. It is frequently used as a treatment modality for patients with aplastic anaemia and other immune disorders. 'Even with leukemias, significant long-term survivals occur in recipients of HLA-compatible marrow' (Kirkpatrick, 1987:2999), especially if transplantation is performed early enough or during remission. Bone marrow transplantation is also being evaluated as a method for the correction of certain genetically determined diseases, such as Hodgkin's disease, and other inborn errors of metabolism.

Since 1970 approximately 9,000 bone marrow transplants have been performed in the world. Throughout the latter half of the 1980s there has been a one-year success rate of about 50 per cent, and improvements are under way. It has been estimated that in the USA some 25,000 potential recipients could benefit from bone marrow transplants, and whilst no figures as yet exist for Europe, a similar number might be expected to benefit (Report of the Conference of European Health Ministers, 1987).

The main problem with bone marrow transplants is that of finding a suitable match in a relatively small donor pool. Bone marrow transplants are only successful with HLA-compatible donors, and the mortality associated with the procedure remains appreciable, with graft versus host disease being the principal complication (ibid). To increase the size of the donor pool registries of HLA-typed donors have been set up in Europe and the USA, and moves towards a European registry look likely to solve the problem of the small size of national pools. Likewise the anticipated developments of banks of genetic material from established bone marrow donors will make a significant contribution to the increase in supply and reduction of costs.

Ovaries and testicles have been transplanted since the 1970s. The first pregnancy following a transplanted ovary took place in Buenos Aires in 1971. In cases of pregnancy following ovary transplant the genetic characteristics of the baby will be those of the woman who donated the ovary, not the mother. Research is currently under way for transplants of foetal ovarian tissue in order to enable women who have entered the menopause in their twenties and thirties to have children. The idea is for viable foetal ovarian tissue to be transplanted into a woman with no functioning ovaries, and if it grows, receiving blood supply from the woman, then pregnancy could be achieved after the menopause. The first testicle transplant was from an identical twin in 1978, to a brother who was born without any testicles. After the operation the man was capable of fathering children.

In recent years there have also been developments in multi-organ transplants, such as heart-lung and liver-pancreas. Heart-lung transplants are usually performed for patients with terminal pulmonary hypertension. The first was at Stanford University in 1981. It is still regarded as an experimental procedure, with only a 50 per cent one-year survival rate (New York Task Force, 1988:17). Apart from medical complications there are other problems: it is hard to find suitable donors; and following brain death there is a quick deterioration of the lungs, so rapid transplantation is essential.

Plans are well under way for a significant extension to programmes involving multi-organ transplants. Since 1985 the transplant centre at the Presbyterian University Hospital in Pittsburgh have been considering plans for 'a simultaneous transplantation of a liver, spleen, stomach, pancreas, and large intestine into one patient in a single operation' (Jonsen, 1988:232).

Perhaps the ultimate in transplant surgery would be the whole body transplant. Now whole body transplants have a long history in the horror/science-fiction genre, from Mary Shelley's *Frankenstein* onwards. But this proposal has been taken seriously by Professor Robert J. White of the University of Cleveland. White has transplanted the brains of dogs into other dogs, and in 1970 transplanted the head of one monkey to the body of another. In later experiments he kept alive two severed monkey heads for a week (White, 1983). Under these conditions, according to White, the animal's brain was able to retain a state of consciousness and response to external stimuli (White, 1983:115–16). In one case, following the transplant of the entire cephalon of a monkey, White records:

> In the ensuing hours following surgery, a complete awake state supervened and, through the available cranial nerve function, the preparation did respond appropriately to external stimulation! It was obvious that the animals could see and did appreciate movement and, indeed, would track with their eyes objects of interest placed in their visual fields. Responsivity to ordinary stimulation was obvious in that, if a loud sound was produced, the cephalon evidenced a facial expression of discomfort. Light pin pricks of the facial tissue, likewise, gave evidence of discomfort on the part of the animal.
>
> These preparations could and did masticate and swallow food, as well as appropriately handling fluids employing the expected muscle movements of tongue and oral cavity. Indeed, one had the impression that the animals were 'hungry and thirsty' and underwent the oral processing of food and liquid with alacrity.
>
> (ibid:117)

To sustain an animal to these conditions did require massive intensive care, and whatever reservations one might have concerning the quality of life of these unfortunate creatures, there is little doubt that they survived the transplant. Nevertheless, these transplanted heads could not control their bodies, as it is impossible to connect between 100 and 200 million severed nerve ends. Yet according to White, 'there is every reason to contemplate that, with additional advances and redesign in surgical and instrumentation technology, similar operations could be performed in the human' (ibid:120). This, of course, is a long way off and techniques may never be perfected, even if such work was ethically permissible. 'These patients' says White, 'would require an incredible army of monitoring and maintenance equipment, as well as a continually available cadre of specially trained physicians and nurses' (ibid:126). Although he does suggest that this would be within the range of 'financial and medical requirements that were found to be necessary for sustaining Dr (Barney) Clark's existence', when he was hospitalized for 112 days following the implantation of an artificial heart (ibid:127). Given White's expectation that consciousness would be retained in the situation involving a human body transplant, the outcome would, on the most optimistic prognosis, resemble that of a quadriplegic person without movement or sensation below the neck, but with limited abilities to hear, see, and with some assistance speak.

In lectures, and on a TV programme (BBC, 8 February 1989), White posed the following scenario concerning whole body transplants. It involves a brilliant scientist whose brain can undoubtedly benefit mankind, but whose body is being destroyed by a virulent form of cancer. This scientist, suggests White, could be the recipient of the body of a donor who has died as the result of massive head injuries. Given the possibility of such a case, however technologically remote, it raises fundamental philosophical and ethical issues which go beyond anything previously considered in bioethics.

It is frequently pointed out that despite life-saving and prolonging benefits, transplantation of kidneys, hearts and livers do not fully restore health, but 'substitute(s) the side-effects of immunosuppressive drugs and a life-long battle against organ rejection for the underlying disease' (New York Task Force, 1988:viii). One transplant surgeon has described renal transplantation, when successful, as giving the patient a 'holiday from dialysis'.

Though not a cure, transplantation provides hope, but with this hope comes fear and anxiety about rejection. There are many who find this too much of a burden, especially when transplantation is conducted in experimental stages. But hope, often against all odds, is part of the human condition. There is a story of a peasant found guilty of stealing a horse which belonged to the King. When sentenced to death he put forward the following plea: 'If you spare my life, I promise that I will teach your horse to talk.' The King accepted the plea, giving the man a year to achieve this task, after which, if he was unsuccessful, the execution would take place. When it was pointed out that he had little chance of teaching the horse to talk, and that the King would surely execute him, the peasant replied: 'In a year a lot may happen; I might die, the King might die, or the horse might learn to talk. But the alternative is my immediate death.' Our peasant has a difficult, and very likely an impossible task. But like those who undergo transplant surgery, he recognizes that it's the only game in town.

The history of organ transplantation is, at one level, a record of scientific and technical success. It is also a history of anxiety and serious moral questioning, which reflects a dialectical movement between the ethical problems of risky and expensive experiments on the one hand and routine therapy using scarce resources on the other. The early renal transplants and cardiac transplants were experimental and raised serious ethical questions about the physician–patient relationship, especially when the likelihood of success was low. In the experimental stage there are serious problems of consent. To what extent are those who consent fully informed? To what extent do they understand what they have consented to? Dr Christian Barnard told Louis Washinsky's wife that he had an '80 per cent chance', which in 1968 was hopelessly unrealistic (New York Task Force, 1988:10). Would it have made any difference to her consent if the odds had been presented more realistically? For some, it clearly would. Prolonging an inevitable dying process has no ethical justification. Yet for others, if there is hope, despite the odds, then experiment is justified. There are no intuitively obvious ethical guidelines here, excepting a prohibition of consent to experimentation based on false expectations.

Yet as experiment gives way to routine therapy, there is the problem of when a surgeon should cease to be an experimenter and become a clinician. Is it when surgical technique is perfected, and when immunosuppressive drugs overcome rejection? But then immunosuppressive regimens can be experimental and some side-effects are still subjects of research. Moreover, with the new role of clinician come fresh moral problems, as the dialectic moves on from the ethics of high risk to the equitable procurement and allocation of the organs and therapeutic resources. For as renal and cardiac transplantation becomes routine, the problems of procurement and allocation loom large. These problems cannot be confined within the discourse of medical professionals; they raise issues of fundamental social concern. There is a need for a governmental role, and responsible media, if efforts to increase procurement and allocation are to be based on equitable grounds. There is a need for public funding, in both the experimental and clinical aspects of transplant surgery. But it is not merely a question of spending the public's money; it is also a question of persuading the public to donate their organs. This highlights greater need for informed public participation in debates on organ transplantation, and a need for analysis of the parameters of ethical concern as a

22

prelude to public guidelines in the form of statutes, quasi-legis-
lation and international agreements.

2

ORGAN TRANSPLANTS AND CRITERIA FOR DEATH

It would be preferable by far for man's future survival to have to abandon transplantation than to agree to remove vital organs from individuals who are not really dead.
(Report of the Conference of European Health Ministers, 1987)

THE MEANING OF DEATH

In the summer of 1978 John Smith, a 45-year-old computer programmer from Minneapolis, and his second wife, Lucy, were touring in Southern California in a car which they had hired for their honeymoon. The freeway accident involved three cars and a truck. Lucy, who was driving, suffered the full impact of the collision and sustained head and chest injuries of such magnitude that it was obvious that she had been killed instantly. John was flung clear of the wreck but sustained massive head injuries and was taken within minutes of the collision to the emergency room of the nearby university hospital. He required several transfusions and a ventilator to maintain oxygenation, although his heart and kidneys appeared to be undamaged.

After 36 hours John was still unconscious and unable to maintain spontaneous respiration. An EEG scan revealed no brain activity and further tests revealed absence of spontaneous motion and no reaction to painful stimuli. It was discovered that John was in possession of a Uniform Anatomical Gift Card and the transplant team were notified and put on alert whilst a search was undertaken to locate John's nearest living kin. This proved futile. After consulting two other physicians and conducting tests which revealed complete absence of brainstem functions, the attending

24

physician declared John dead despite the fact that his heart and lungs were functioning with mechanical assistance. He then made a decision to move John to the operating room where his heart, lungs, and kidneys were transplanted into two other patients.

Three days later Joseph Smith, John's son from his first marriage, arrived at the hospital, followed closely by Lucy's sister, Mary. Both were overcome with grief which later turned to anger. In due course they initiated legal proceedings.

Joseph's attorney argued several points: that Minnesota, John's State, did not recognize brain death and that his father was alive at the time his organs were removed. He argued that under Minnesotan law the remains of the deceased belong to the next of kin, namely Joseph. He argued that the hospital should not have appointed a member of the transplant team to be John's attending physician, since his allegiance appeared to be directed towards the patients requiring organs rather than to John. The hospital countered that death occurred in California, not Minnesota, and that John was pronounced dead in accord with local laws which did recognize brain death. Moreover, the hospital maintained that John's donor card expressed a clear indication of his wishes, and that his death had been determined objectively and confirmed by two other physicians.

The arguments pressed by the attorney representing Lucy's sister came later and were directed at John and Lucy's testamentary dispositions. It transpired that in the event of Lucy predeceasing John the whole of her estate would pass to John. On the other hand, according to the terms of John's will, on his demise all of his estate would pass to his son, Joseph. In the event of a simultaneous death the joint estates would be divided equally between Joseph and Mary. Mary's attorney argued that John and Lucy met their deaths simultaneously and that John's body was artificially maintained until his organs were transplanted. In reply, Joseph's attorney argued that John had survived Lucy until the moment artificial ventilation was terminated and his heart and lungs removed. The ensuing legal battle turned on matters of clinical facts which were themselves determined by the conceptual significance of the relevant criteria for death: in other words, on what it *means* to be dead.

The philosophical nature of the issues raised in the above example can be seen more clearly if the following questions are addressed:

25

(i) At the time John's organs were removed, was he dead or alive?

(ii) Who died first, John or Lucy?

These two questions refer to philosophical beliefs concerning what it means to be dead, and also to the particular concept of death employed. They also refer to matters of clinical fact which are connected with the ethical and legal issues.

(iii) Would John have been considered dead or alive in this country at the time his organs were removed? Upon what evidence should the answer be based? What would his status have been in other countries, in other religious traditions?

(iv) What is it that is lost in death that causes us to regard the person we have known as 'gone'? Is it spontaneous breathing and heartbeat, consciousness, cognition, or characteristics associated with speech, reason, and similar traits that marked him or her as a living person? Or is it an entity such as a spirit or soul that has departed? Which of these should we choose, or which combination should we choose, or what other feature or features might be included?

It must be stressed that unless death is defined then attempts to verify it empirically will be meaningless. Technical data cannot provide answers to what are essentially metaphysical and moral questions. Criteria for death, and arguments about more reliable tests for death, must be related to some overall concept of what death means. For at stake here are our notions of 'personhood', 'humanity', 'life', and the moral respect accorded to a living being. Quite obviously these questions raise issues which transcend judgements concerning clinical facts, for they involve a whole background of metaphysical, moral, political, and legal considerations which ultimately relate to what is *meant* by death.

One of the reasons why these conceptual issues have come to the foreground is that developments in the biomedical sciences have disrupted the belief that death is a momentary event characterized by the simultaneous cessation of all characteristics associated with life. Loss of consciousness, respiration, heartbeat, circulation, and failure of other vital systems are no longer necessarily simultaneous events. Since many of the traditional 'signs' of life may be prolonged indefinitely, it has now become a matter of both practical and moral necessity to develop a definition of death (primarily a philosophical task) from which criteria and tests for death can be logically derived (primarily an empirical task).

For most of us, our early knowledge about dying was influenced by novels, films, and television. Enemy soldiers, villains, Red Indians, cowboys, and gangsters died in a simple straightforward way. They toppled like trees. If an attempt was made to confirm death, it consisted of listening for a heartbeat or touching the wrist to determine a pulse. Occasionally, a glass might be held close to the mouth to ascertain absence of respiration. As a rule, sick or old people remained lucid until the end, before expiring in front of relatives who recognized death before the doctor shook his head, drew over the sheets, and signed the death certificate. This scene, so familiar in films, is vastly different from death in a modern ICU, where none of the traditional criteria would be regarded as both necessary and sufficient for a diagnosis of death, suspension of therapy, and possible authorization of organ removal.

Contemporary western culture expresses a need to be better informed about death, which is not unconnected with the vast array of technology employed to monitor and possibly prolong the dying process. At one time death and dying were considered to be very personal experiences, but media exposure in recent years reflects a different attitude. Television crews interview dying victims of various diseases and close-up shots of distressed relatives appear frequently on news bulletins and in documentaries. Executions have been televised and fatal motorway accidents feature in peak-viewing TV serials. This cultural fascination with death suggests that some of the conceptual problems raised in recent debates about the end-points of life are only in part a response to the biomedical revolution of the past twenty years. Rather, the technology itself is a response to a deeper moral concern with the meaning of death. Brain death might well be a technical concept arising out of modern science, but the research out of which this concept has emerged reflects a growing cultural fascination with the subject of death in all its guises. For decades it was considered proper that the definition and criteria for death were strictly a medical matter, but in an era of organ transplants and resuscitation technology, new definitions have emerged and the arguments generated by proponents of these new definitions extend enquiries into the meaning of death beyond the boundaries of medicine, and in some cases require public participation in the form of legal guidelines and directives.

The perplexity about death in current discussions about organ transplants must be seen in this light, for it is indicative of the public's need to be better informed about the process of dying and its possible postponement. Whereas formerly physicians accepted death as a natural phenomenon, but strove to eliminate certain diseases which caused death, there is nowadays a tendency to regard death itself as a disease to be eliminated by medical science. Physicians and medical researchers frequently allow themselves to be portrayed as front-line troops in a war against death itself. The vast array of technology and expertise employed to monitor and postpone death should not be seen as medical science out of control – as it is so often portrayed. Contemporary sophisticated health care technology no doubt contributes to, but is also in response to, a deeper moral concern to extend the boundaries of life. Transplant technology, along with other developments in medical science, is in part a response to changing cultural attitudes about death and medicine itself. This attitude is captured by Carse (1978:324):

> Death is not a limit within which we are to develop our humanity, according to this view, but the very enemy that robs us of our humanity, and therefore an enemy that must be destroyed in the interests of rescuing that humanity. It is no accident that we speak of 'fighting' an epidemic or 'hunting out and conquering' the cause of a crippling disease. The medical profession is not a public service subvened to make our lives more pleasant; it is an army we are determined to train and equip well enough to be sure it will win. Responsible medical scientists are already speaking freely of the time in which all disease will be vanquished, and a large part of the public's fascination with DNA research surely rises from that tiny possibility that someone will pull the winning ticket in the genetic lottery and offer us all eternal youth.

This change in cultural attitudes has accompanied a shift of emphasis in theoretical and practical questions associated with death. For the Greeks and early Chinese the acceptance of death as a natural event meant that greater emphasis could be placed on speculations regarding the possibility of some kind of spiritual life

28

after death. In a secular age there is more concern with the mechanics of death, its postponement, and the possible reversal of the dying process. The transplantation of vital organs, such as heart and lungs, has nevertheless reintroduced a sense of religious awe, in the reflection that life can be saved through death.

Although the definition of death is not strictly a medical matter, and is influenced by philosophical and religious considerations, society nevertheless recognizes the authority of physicians in this area. For this reason the following investigation into the meaning of death will be arbitrarily restricted to judgements about death in clinical contexts. Thus quasi-legal concepts, such as 'missing presumed dead', or concepts of death in terms of the subject's alienation from civil society, will not be addressed here.

IRREVERSIBILITY

Inherent in any medically grounded definition of death is the assumption that death is an irreversible state which involves irreversible loss of respiratory and neural functions. Normally, it is assumed that death occurs at a specific time, although from a biological standpoint it can be considered as a more gradual process.

If an irreversible loss is central to the concept of death, then it follows that if a patient were to recover after being pronounced dead, it should not be said that he or she was dead but is now alive again, but rather that he or she was alive all the time. For this reason when dealing with accounts of patients who have allegedly returned from death – despite well documented evidence of near death experiences (NDEs) and out of body experiences (OBEs) – one is only dealing with highly dramatized descriptions of certain states associated with the loss of consciousness during temporary cardiac arrest (see Woodhouse, 1987:1–18). The fact that similarities between so many reported NDEs and OBEs have not been adequately explained does not provide evidence of the reversibility of death.

There are, of course, religious views which reflect the belief that death does not involve total extinction; that there is everlasting life for those who have not accepted the wages of sin; that the candle burns in some other sense after it has been extinguished. To emphasize these beliefs many religions portray death as either a transition or a journey. Sometimes food is placed at the side of

29

the corpse to sustain the traveller. But none of these practices and beliefs actually contradict a definition of death which is expressed in terms of the irreversible cessation of vital functions. When the ancient Egyptians and early Chinese left bowls of food for the deceased they would have been as surprised as any twentieth-century physician if the corpse had managed to consume it. For these practices never entailed a prediction that life would return to the corpse, and it was recognized that death necessarily involved an irreversible interruption of physical continuity. The metaphorical attribution of physical wants and needs, which is displayed in numerous religious practices, should be seen as a way of showing respect for the life that has passed, not as a crude prediction concerning the future physical state of the being that was.

What is irreversibly lost in death?

When answering this question it is important to avoid the use of vague and undetermined concepts. Consider a definition such as 'Death is the loss of that which is essentially significant to a human being'. This is clearly unsatisfactory, for we can say that 'this patient has lost what is essentially significant but is still alive'. Concepts like 'essentially significant' are inherently undetermined and should be avoided unless further guidelines are provided. For example, it could be argued that 'massive brain damage' or 'loss of reproductive functions', the loss of a film star's physical attractiveness, or a radical departure from one's moral principles, might constitute necessary and sufficient grounds for the judgement that what is 'essentially significant' has been lost. If 'the loss of that which is essentially significant' is to have any physiological meaning as a concept of death, then it must be so framed that it describes a state where the organism as a whole cannot function. This is why brain death has been proposed as a definition of death which surpasses traditional cardio-respiratory concepts.

The only wholly satisfactory definition of death is one which trumps other concepts insofar as it yields a diagnosis of death that is beyond dispute. It is both morally and theoretically unacceptable to rest satisfied with a situation where there are competing formulations of death, or for a patient to be pronounced dead according to one definition but alive according to another. Any criterion which, when fulfilled, left it possible to say that the patient was still alive, would be unsatisfactory. For this reason, definitions of death which specifically relate to the loss of moral, spiritual, or cognitive aspects alone, would be inadequate.

So far it has been argued that any valid concept of death must be necessarily linked to an irreversible physical change in the state of the organism as a whole. Given the potential reversibility of states associated with traditional cardio-respiratory concepts, only a brain-related concept can provide both necessary and sufficient criteria for the death of the organism as a whole. But being brain dead is not an alternative way of being dead: brain death is a reformulation of the traditional concept according to which loss of heartbeat and circulation is not a state of death in itself, but is an indication (in certain cases where ventilatory support is absent) of the imminence of death. That is to say, according to the brain-related concept of death, former criteria, such as loss of respiration, heartbeat, and pulse, acquire a different status. They are indicators regarding the state of the brain. For the patient is alive until the brain is dead.

Nevertheless, the precise formulation of the concept of brain death has continued to generate philosophical, ethical, legal, and medical controversy. The clarification of the conceptual grounds in this controversy is primarily a philosophical task, but in order to do so it is necessary to examine the development of the concept of brain death over the past twenty or so years before addressing the issue of brain death in a broader cultural context.

BRAIN DEATH: DEVELOPMENT OF THE CONCEPT AND CRITERIA

Until the early 1960s and the advent of techniques for taking over the functions of the lungs and heart, the public had shown almost complete acceptance of medical practice concerning the diagnosis of death. This has not always been the case. Distrust of the profession's competence had been evident in scores of pamphlets and tracts written in the eighteenth and nineteenth centuries (Arnold *et al.*, 1968). In 1740 it had been suggested by Jacques Bénigne Winslow that putrefaction was the only sure sign of death. Such a proposal reflected a total loss of public confidence in their doctors. Yet putrefaction has never been seriously advanced as a definition of death by either physicians or philosophers.

The prestige of physicians increased, however, during the

mid-nineteenth century as health care sought to become more scientific and professional, although distrust of the kind expressed in Edgar Allan Poe's novel, *The Tell-Tale Heart*, continued throughout the century. Nevertheless, the development of certain technological aids, such as the stethoscope, enabled a more accurate detection of heartbeat and respiration, and was an important factor in the growth of public confidence in the ability to diagnose death. In the twentieth century scepticism has returned in some areas (Browne, 1983). It will be argued that this scepticism is without foundation, and that refinements in diagnostic criteria have reached the point where public acceptance is justified.

The earliest references in the neurological literature to states resembling brain death go back to the 1890s. In 1898 Sir Dyce Duckworth reported on four cases with structural brain lesions in which 'the function of respiration had earlier ceased for some hours before that of the circulation' (Duckworth, 1898:145). Then in 1902 Harvey Cushing described a patient whose spontaneous respiration ceased as a result of an intracranial tumour, but whose heart was kept beating for 23 hours with artificial respiration (Black, 1978:395).

The concept of brain death really emerged in France, in 1959. Early that year a group of French neurosurgeons described a condition which they termed, 'death of the central nervous system' (Jouvet, 1959:805). The characteristics of this state were 'persistent apnoeic coma, absent brainstem and tendon reflexes, and an electrically silent brain'. These patients had no detectable electrophysiological activity in either the superficial or deeper parts of their brains (Wertheimer *et al.*, 1959:87). Whilst they looked like cadavers a regular pulse could be discerned as long as ventilation was maintained. Although the authors did not address the issue of whether this state was equivalent to death, they concluded that the persistence of this condition for 18 to 24 hours warranted disconnection from the ventilator. Later that year a more complete account of the condition was published by two Parisian neurologists, Mollaret and Goulon, (1959) who called it *coma dépassé* (a state beyond coma). They were not prepared to equate *coma dépassé* with death and, unlike their predecessors, they did not advocate the withdrawal of ventilatory support. The patients had all sustained massive, irreversible, structural brain damage. Patients in a state of *coma dépassé* were in a state of irreversible coma associated with an irreversible loss of the capacity to breathe.

32

They had not only lost all capacity to respond to external stimuli, they could not even cope with their internal milieu: they were poikilothermic, had diabetes insipidus, and could not sustain their own blood pressure. The cardiac prognosis of this condition was at most a few days, but sometimes as little as a few hours (Pallis, 1983:34).

Outside France the term *coma dépassé* never really caught on. The condition was of course encountered wherever resuscitation was sufficiently well organized, and intensive care units adequately equipped, to prevent irreversible apnoea immediately resulting in cessation of cardiac action. During this period there was no attempt to relate observations of this condition to any well-founded concept of death. Neither of the two French groups discussed the meaning of death (which is probably why they suggested different courses of action for what was essentially the same condition). By the late 1960s an increasing rate of organ transplantation and greater successes in resuscitation provided a background to the need for greater philosophical clarity concerning what it meant to be dead. The lack of such clarity was reflected in the ambiguous and often confusing terminology used at that time. The term 'irreversible coma' was sometimes employed to refer to a condition which was equivalent to '*coma dépassé*'. The term 'brain death' referred to the same state. Although the terminology was in a state of flux, the construct 'brain death' achieved a degree of precision that allowed it to be used in a popular way (Korein, 1978). The term *coma dépassé* survived in France until 24 May 1988 when it was rejected in favour of 'brain death' by the French Academy of Medicine, who commented that their decision 'ends semantic ambiguity which leads to clinical ambiguity' (*Le Monde*, 27 May 1988).

In 1968 the Ad Hoc Committee of the Harvard Medical School to Examine the Definition of Brain Death published its report, and brain death (which was exactly what the French had described as *coma dépassé*) achieved world-wide recognition (Ad Hoc Committee of the Harvard Medical School, 1968). The Harvard criteria for brain death were fourfold:

(1) absence of cerebral responsiveness;
(2) absence of induced or spontaneous movement;
(3) absence of spontaneous respiration;
(4) absence of brainstem and deep tendon reflexes.

An isoelectric EEG was deemed to be of 'great confirmatory value' but the performance of an EEG was not considered mandatory. The report specified two conditions which were capable of mimicking the state of brain death and which had to be excluded in each case: hypothermia and drug intoxication. Finally, the report recommended that tests be repeated over a period of 24 hours to document the persistence of the condition. Since then numerous patients throughout the world have been diagnosed as brain dead, maintained on ventilators and observed until their hearts stopped. No patient meeting the Harvard criteria has ever recovered despite the most heroic management.

THE BRAINSTEM FORMULATION

In the years following the publication of the Harvard Report it was gradually realized that the clinically testable component of brain death was death of the brainstem (*brainstem death*). In 1971 the work of two neurosurgeons, Mohandas and Chou, in Minneapolis, had a profound influence on thinking and practice regarding the diagnosis of death on neurological grounds. From detailed observations of patients who had sustained massive intra-cranial damage they concluded that irreversible damage to the brainstem was 'the point of no return' in the dying process, and that a diagnosis of this state 'could be based on clinical judgement' (Mohandas and Chou, 1971:211–18). Their recommendations became known as the Minnesota criteria, which were significant in that they introduced aetiological preconditions to the diagnosis of brain death. A valid diagnosis of a dead brainstem, they held, was context-dependent in the sense that an essential precondition was knowledge of 'irreparable intracranial lesions'.

This point about context-dependency has not been fully appreci-ated by critics of brainstem death in the popular media, who frequently assume that tests are conducted in ignorance of the cause of the coma. Later guidelines stress that the all-important characteristic of irreversibility can only be established with refer-ence to crucial preconditions. Not only must there be a known primary diagnosis which accounts for the cause of the coma, there must also be evidence that all reversible causes of brainstem dysfunction (such as hypothermia and drug intoxication) have been excluded. This, of course, may take time, which is why it is misleading to speak simply of tests for brainstem death.

In a detailed account of the essential steps involved in the diagnosis of brainstem death, Pallis (1989) stresses the importance of an 'unhurried approach' with an attitude that ventilation of the comatose patient should continue 'for as long as it takes to ascertain that the preconditions have been met, and that all conditions that have to be excluded have been excluded'. When it is deemed appropriate to conduct tests the objective is to (a) ascertain the absence of cardinal brainstem reflexes and (b) rigorously document apnoea. These procedures involve a battery of clinical tests (each reinforcing the information to be derived from the others), such that the determination of death does not depend on a single procedure or the assessment of a single function. It is therefore wholly misleading to compare the expression 'brainstem death' with expressions which refer to the loss of a single organ such as the heart or the liver. When properly understood 'brainstem death' does not signify the death of an organ; it is the point at which the individual no longer functions as an integrated being. This entails the irreversible loss of the capacity for consciousness together with the irreversible loss of the capacity for respiration and integrated organic functioning.

The significance of brainstem criteria can be appreciated with reference to its contribution to the continuous function of the organism as a whole. In its upper part the brainstem contains crucial centres for generating the capacity for consciousness. Thus whilst extensive damage to the cortex, from trauma or anoxia, may not cause permanent unconsciousness, there is one functional unit without whose activity consciousness cannot exist. This is the ascending reticular activating system, or ARAS, which is situated in the upper part of the brainstem. Acute, strategically situated bilateral lesions in the paramedian tegmental area of the rostral brainstem entail loss of the capacity for consciousness. In the lower part of the brainstem are mechanisms which control the respiratory centre. Thus lesions of critical areas in the lower part of the brainstem are associated with the permanent cessation of the ability to breathe which in turn deprives the heart and cerebral hemispheres of oxygen, causing them to cease functioning. It is death of the brainstem (which in practice is nearly always the result of a massive increase in intracranial pressure) which produces the crucial signs (apnoeic coma with absent brainstem reflexes) which doctors detect at the bedside, when they diagnose brain death.

Detailed research into the nature and functions of the brainstem is a fairly recent phenomenon and no doubt much more has still to be learnt. But there is a sense in which loss of brainstem functions has always been equated with death. Throughout history humans have executed their unfortunate fellows by means of hanging or decapitating, thus recognizing death as the severance of brain from the body. Even large carnivores recognize brainstem death, since they seize upon and shake their prey, inflicting atlanto-axial dislocation and brainstem death in their victims (Pallis, 1989).

Since irreversible loss of brainstem function necessarily involves loss of both the capacity for consciousness and the capacity to breathe, a very strong case can be made for linking brainstem death to traditional philosophical and religious-based definitions of death as 'the departure of the soul from the body' and 'loss of the breath of life'. In a very important sense brainstem death does not involve a new definition of death, but is a definition which has replaced uncertainty. For when properly understood, irreversible loss of brainstem functions has always provided the mechanism of death.

The last twenty years have seen the gradual acceptance of the proposition that death of the brain is the necessary and sufficient condition for the death of the individual. The last decade has seen a parallel development: the gradual realization that death of the brainstem is the necessary and sufficient condition for the death of the brain as a whole – and that brainstem death is therefore itself synonymous with death of the individual. This latter realization received implicit recognition in statements issued by the Conference of Medical Royal Colleges and their faculties in the UK in 1976 and 1979. Proponents of brainstem criteria for death argue that death of the brainstem is itself death (a philosophical position). They also point out that a diagnosis of brainstem death has in every observed case been followed by eventual circulatory arrest (an empirical observation).

THE WHOLE ORGANISM OR THE ORGANISM AS A WHOLE?

Any valid concept of death must necessarily be linked to an irreversible change in the state of the organism as a whole. Life depends on the integration of physiological functions such as

36

ingestion, digestion, absorption, respiration, distribution (circu-lation), metabolism, excretion, and egestion or elimination. The concept of the irreversible loss of function of the organism as a whole implies the irreversible loss of this integrated functioning. In these purely biological respects the death of a man or a woman is no different to the death of a dog, for what is lost in death is the ability to integrate and organize component systems. Essential to the maintenance of the organ as a whole is the role of a critical system which organizes and integrates other systems and which cannot be replaced by an artifact (Lamb, 1985:33–40). This critical system is the brain, whose integrating function depends on an intact brainstem. The brainstem can be thought of as the critical system of the critical system, without whose function the organism as a whole could not survive as an independent biological entity. Pallis (1983:3) has described brainstem death as the 'physiological kernel' of brain death. Since destruction of the brainstem precludes integrated functioning of the brain as a whole, a diagnosis of irreversible loss of brainstem function is the quintessence of whole brain death. In the overwhelming majority of cases brainstem death is not a primary event. It is the ultimate pathological reper-cussion of processes above the tentorium [the tentorium is a fibrous ring which separates the cerebral hemispheres (above) from the cerebellum and brainstem (below)] which cause massive increases in intracranial pressure. A concept of brainstem death yields unambiguous clinical criteria which can be objectively tested. It is both clinically and conceptually superior to traditional heart-related concepts. It is also superior to dualistic formulations which, by offering a choice between brain- or heart-related cri-teria, cannot be said to be derived from any well-founded concept of death.

The clearly identifiable state of brainstem death should not be confused with another clinically, ontologically, and philosophi-cally, very different condition in which massive brain damage is largely confined to the cerebral hemispheres, sparing much of the brainstem and in particular the capacity to breathe spontaneously. This is the *persistent vegetative state*. Such patients have usually been the victims of severe head injury or anoxic insults to the brain (lack of oxygen wrecks the cerebral hemispheres before it destroys the brainstem). Such patients may be found in institutions for the chronically sick all over the world. It is important, both scientifically and ethically, to avoid confusing brainstem death

37

with such non-cognitive states. Patients in persistent vegetative states are said to be 'awake but not aware' (Jennett and Plum, 1972). They display no evidence of self-awareness and exhibit no purposeful response to external stimuli. Their eyes may open periodically, and they show sleep–wake sequences. They may exhibit yawning and chewing movements and may swallow spontaneously. A variety of simple or complex reflex responses may be elicited from them. Unlike brainstem death (which signifies the 'death of the organism as a whole' and has a cardiac prognosis seldom exceeding a week), the persistent vegetative state has a potential cardiac prognosis of months or even years.

The appropriate formulation of the concept of 'brainstem death' is 'the irreversible loss of function of the organism as a whole' (Lamb, 1985). This is not the same as 'death of the whole organism', i.e. of every one of its cells. This latter formulation is often implied – although unstated – in arguments which maintain that the concept of death should be left undetermined, or that death is a process with no special point at which a non-arbitrary diagnosis can be factually ascertained (Morison, 1971; Browne, 1983). Whereas criteria for 'the irreversible loss of function of the organism as a whole' (brainstem death) require simple and straightforward tests, criteria for the 'death of the whole organism' could only be met by tests for putrefaction, for cellular life in certain tissues may continue long after the organism as a whole has ceased to function.

The argument that death should remain undefined has no place in a world where practical decisions are needed. Criteria for 'the irreversible loss of function of the organism as a whole' can be determined with precision, and appropriate diagnostic tests have been developed (Pallis, 1983; 1989). The concept of death so defined presupposes the irreversible loss of the capacity for consciousness and the irreversible loss of the capacity to breathe, and hence to sustain a spontaneous heartbeat. It supersedes (or some would say merely reformulates in secular terms) ethical and religious-based concepts. Its basis is the death of the critical system as measured by tests for the irreversible loss of brainstem function.

BRAINSTEM DEATH IN A BROADER CULTURAL CONTEXT

The brainstem concept of death stresses both the irreversible loss of the capacity for consciousness and loss of the capacity for

38

spontaneous respiration. In this respect it is compatible with older beliefs about death in various cultures and religious traditions.

Although there are numerous cultural attitudes towards the dying and the dead, the more basic similarities between these attitudes outweigh the differences. Human beings are the only species to manifest moral respect for the dead; the only species to dispose of the dead in a systematic way, and the only species to give a meaning to death. In most religions the meaning of death has been bound up with notions of an after-life, or some form of continued existence. But whatever meaning was given to death, the fact of death was accepted as an empirical matter, not requiring precise definition or further elaboration. Death was – as most dictionaries still define it – the end of life, ceasing to be. But technological intervention in the dying process has necessitated a requirement for a philosophical, ethical, and clinically applicable, secular equivalent to religious concepts which were often formulated in terms of the departure of the soul or loss of the breath of life.

In Western Europe, from earliest records, the traditional view was that death occurred when the soul departed with the last breath of life. It was only after circulation was discovered in the 17th century and ausculation was introduced in 1819 that absence of heartbeat was seen as a sign of death. It would seem, in this respect, that the brainstem formulation of death with its emphasis on irreversible apnoea, is compatible with traditional beliefs. This, of course, is not to say that early beliefs were formulated with a brainstem definition in mind. One of the basic problems to be faced when examining the significance of brain-related concepts of death for various religions is that most religious creeds evolved at a time when little was known about medicine and biology. Moreover, in earlier times the procedure for establishing death was non-controversial; the main concern was with coming to terms with death and the possibility of surviving it in some extra-worldly state. Whereas the early Egyptians saw the heart as the vital organ and appeared to place little emphasis upon the brain, in Talmudic sources absence of heartbeat was never considered an essential aspect in the determination of death. Orthodox Jewish teachings identified the decapitated state with death. The Code of Laws was well aware that the state resembling death was beheading; the agonized cries of a decapitated man were looked upon as an aftermath of death. Thus in the Babylonian Talmud (Tractate

Chulin: 21 A) it stressed that 'the death throws of a decapitated man are not signs of life, any more than were the twitchings of a lizard's amputated tail'. Insofar as brainstem death is a neurological equivalent to decapitation it follows that the brainstem concept is perfectly compatible with Jewish teachings. In the rabbinical literature it is the ability to breathe independently which is the 'esse' of life. This is given greater prominence than the heartbeat. In Genesis 2: 7 it states that: 'the Lord God formed man out of the dust of the ground, and breathed into his nostrils the breath of life; and man became a living soul.' What mattered most, in early Jewish sources, was the capacity to breathe spontaneously, but although apnoea is a necessary condition for death, it is not sufficient. A ventilated patient whose only defect is paralysis of the motor neurons to the muscles responsible for respiration due to neurological disorder is obviously alive despite an inability to breathe spontaneously. Thus in order to provide both necessary and sufficient criteria for death, apnoea would have to be accompanied by other criteria which indicated that sufficient damage to the brain equivalent to physiological decapitation had occurred. This can be observed in the application of brainstem criteria for death which insists upon tests to determine complete loss of physical integration, capacity for consciousness, as well as irreversible apnoea. More recent corroboration of compatibility between criteria for brain death and Judaic beliefs can be seen in the fact that Israel is one of the countries where brain-related criteria for death are now applied.

Some of the more refined tests occasionally advocated for whole brain death might not be so easily integrated with Jewish teaching. Talmudic ethical imperatives stress the infinite value of life, which includes the remaining seconds of a person's life. Hence nothing should be done to shorten that life, not even shaking the bed on which a patient is dying. In this respect certain invasive diagnostic procedures, such as four vessel angiography, would be incompatible with Talmudic imperatives (Pallis, 1987:1037).

In Muslim sources death is repeatedly compared with sleep. The departure of the soul normally takes place during sleep. This emphasis on sleep is compatible with brainstem criteria, according to which tests are conducted on comatose patients. Both Anglican and Roman Catholic belief systems also place emphasis on the separation of the soul from the body, but there seem to be no objections to evidence of this phenomenon being based on neurological grounds. Early Christian sources generally located the soul in the head, which is why they endorsed double baptism for two-headed monsters. The Papal address of Pius XII raised the question whether in ICUs doctors might be 'continuing resuscitation despite the fact that the soul may have left the body'. But he left the actual determination of death to the physicians. So far there have been no official pronouncements on brainstem death from any of the Christian churches, but most of the leading moral theologians have accepted criteria for death based on neurological grounds.

The traditional Roman Catholic understanding of death is in relation to the moment the soul leaves the body. Since what actually happens at this moment is not an observable phenomenon, death is acknowledged in relation to physically determinable signs which indicate apparent death. Signs such as cessation of heartbeat and breathing have been traditionally accepted as reasonably accurate indicators of apparent death. In cases where artificial support systems maintain heart and lung function and the brainstem is irreversibly destroyed so that there is no possibility of restoring integrated bodily functions, it would seem that a situation has been reached which produces an even stronger case for recognizing apparent death. The address of Pope Pius XII on the subject of patients who are irreversibly comatose upheld the concept of death in terms of the separation of the soul from the body, but the Pope pointed out that 'in practice one must take into account the lack of precision of the terms "body" and "separation". . . . As to the pronouncement of death in certain particular cases . . . the answer cannot be deduced from religious and moral principle and under this aspect, does not fall within competence of the Church' (Pope Pius XII, 1957:398). The papal point here appears to be that the theological concept of death as the separation of the soul from the body is perfectly compatible with neurological criteria for diagnosing death in cases involving irreversibly comatose states.

The Protestant Churches do not regard the manner of establishing death as a theological issue and have not offered any objections to brain-related criteria. The Report of the Swedish Committee on Defining Death (1984) indicated that representatives of the Church of Sweden and various free churches had no objections to brain-related criteria. Likewise other religions such as Hinduism and Buddhism, and the Greek Orthodox Church, do not specify guidelines concerning the mechanism of death. In Greece, however, brain death criteria have been officially applied since 1978. Although no directives are outlined, some of the African religions assume that death occurs with the cessation of breathing, which is perfectly compatible with criteria for loss of brainstem function. In Japan traditional beliefs equate the heart with the source of the soul and there has been resistance to the concept of brain death. But in 1988 the Life Ethics Council of the Japanese Medical Society accepted that brain death was a valid definition of death, and that patients meeting criteria for brain death could be accepted as cadaver organ donors.

3

THE REDEFINITION ISSUE

... the times have been
That when the brains were out, the man would die,
And there an end.
But now, they rise again.

(Shakespeare, *Macbeth* IV:iii, 78)

INTRODUCTION

This chapter examines proposals that death should be redefined
with criteria for the determination of death based on ontological
grounds; that is, in terms of the loss of personhood or personal
identity so determined in terms of the loss of structures associated
with consciousness and cognition. Exponents of ontological definitions contrast them with biological definitions, such as the brainstem definition, which in the previous chapter was defined as 'the
irreversible loss of function of the organism as a whole'. It will
be argued here that ontological formulations are theoretically
unsatisfactory; that ontological and biological formulations are not
even genuine rival formulations, in the sense that brainstem death
also necessarily entails loss of consciousness and cognition. It will
be argued that the problem with person-oriented definitions is
that (a) they provide an inadequate level of diagnostic certainty,
and (b) even if they were certain it would still leave unanswered
questions of whether tests for the loss of consciousness and cognition could amount to the equivalent of loss of personhood,
and whether indeed loss of personhood was death. This mass of
uncertainty, it will be argued, provides some justification for slippery slope objections to some of the proposed redefinitions
of death.

43

ONTOLOGICAL AND BIOLOGICAL DEFINITIONS

In recent years a greater awareness of the philosophical problems involved in the brain death issue has led to discussions concerning the criteria for loss of personhood, and the proposal that loss of personhood, or personal identity, should be accepted as valid criteria for a determination of death, and hence authorization, where appropriate, of organ removal for transplantation purposes. Definitions appealing to loss of personhood have been described as ontological definitions (Gervais, 1987) which are contrasted with biological definitions expressed in whole brain or brainstem formulations. Those who argue for a redefinition of death based on ontological criteria appeal to the loss of higher brain functions which, so they claim, are characteristic of the persistent vegetative state and various forms of anencephaly. Sometimes ambiguous or misleading synonyms, such as 'cerebral death', 'neocortical death', or the 'apallic syndrome' are used in this context.

A collection of papers, recently published, under the title of *Death: Beyond Whole-Brain Criteria*, put forward the case for personal identity, or higher brain formulations of death (Zaner, 1988). One of the authors outlined the benefits of such a redefinition for the procurement of transplant organs.

> A neocortical death standard could significantly increase availability and access to transplants because patients (including anencephalics) declared dead under a neocortical definition could be biologically maintained for years as opposed to a few hours or days, as in the case of whole brain death. Under the present Uniform Anatomical Gift Act, this raises the possibility that neocortically dead bodies or parts could be donated and maintained for long-term research, as organ banks, or for other purposes such as drug testing or manufacturing biological compounds.
>
> (Smith, 1988:129)

Arguments supporting ontological or higher brain formulations of death are concerned with criteria seeking to describe the minimum necessary qualities for personhood, defined in terms of psychological abilities. It is argued that since the loss of higher brain functions entails the loss of continuous mental processes, then a redefinition of brain death must stress loss of personal identity. Ontological definitions do not attribute any significance

44

to the persistence of other functions such as spontaneous respiration and heartbeat.

In most of the literature on brain death there are references to the higher or lower parts of the brain, which are said to be responsible for cognitive and integrative functions respectively. Ontological definitions are said to focus primarily on the former, whilst biological definitions address the latter. But the situation is not as straightforward as this. Terms such as 'higher' and 'lower' do not have any precise physiological meanings. Among neuroscientists there is general agreement 'that such "higher brain" functions as consciousness and cognition may not be mediated strictly by the cerebral cortex; rather, they probably result from complex interrelations between brainstem and cortex' (President's Commission, 1981:15). Bearing this point in mind the distinction between higher and lower parts of the brain will be maintained in this part of the discussion for convenience and conformity with contemporary usage.

The higher brain, or cerebrum, controls movement and speech. It is concerned with the *content* of consciousness (broadly comprising the sum total of an individual's cognitive and affective endowment). The content of consciousness must be distinguished from the *capacity* for consciousness, which is determined by structures in the brainstem. The upper parts of the brainstem activate the cerebral hemispheres and are responsible for generating the capacity for consciousness. Although the capacity for consciousness (a brainstem function) is not the same as the content of consciousness (a function of the higher brain) it is, nevertheless, an essential precondition of the latter. If there is no brainstem function there can be no cognitive and affective life; no thoughts or feelings, and no social interaction. It should be stressed that the capacity for spontaneous breathing is also a function of the brainstem. Apnoea is thus a necessary, though not a sufficient, sign of a non-functioning brainstem.

Gervais argues for an ontological definition of death according to which 'the permanent absence of consciousness' is a 'measure of human death' (Gervais, 1987:11). She endorses criteria for death based on cessation of neocortical functions. She also includes in this category anencephalic infants and patients in persistent vegetative states. In common with several contributors to *Death: Beyond Whole-Brain Criteria* (Zaner, 1988), Gervais appears to equate neocortical death (a neuropathological concept) with the

45

persistent vegetative state (a clinical concept), although the former is never clearly defined. This kind of confusion is damaging to her case because it illicitly subsumes two very different conditions under the proposed redefinition of death. It should be stressed that criteria fulfilling the concept of neocortical death require an isoelectric EEG. Few patients in persistent vegetative states would fulfil this requirement. Neocortical death is a very rare variant of the persistent vegetative state, as the vast majority of the latter have not suffered anoxic or ischaemical insults of sufficient severity to abolish the EEG. The significance of this distinction between neocortical death and the persistent vegetative state can be appreciated in terms of survival rates. It is simply misleading to describe patients in persistent vegetative states, such as Ms Karen Quinlan, who survived many years and exhibited an EEG reading, as neocortically dead.

Gervais' case in favour of a consciousness-oriented definition of death is advanced on ethical grounds. She criticizes the brainstem formulation of death as presented by Lamb (1978; 1985) because it allegedly rests on purely biological considerations. Lamb, she says, sees death as 'a fact awaiting discovery' (Gervais, 1987:155) whereas her consciousness-oriented definition was 'chosen on the basis of ethical reflection'.

In one important aspect Gervais has not adequately represented the brainstem formulation. It was not advocated on purely empirical grounds, but rather it was stressed, repeatedly, that brainstem death is an ethically superior formulation because, in matters of life and death, objective, testable criteria concerning presence or absence of vital functions, are more reliable than indeterminate assessments concerning the quality of residual life, or speculations regarding personhood, or utilitarian requirements for transplant organs (Lamb, 1985). The whole debate about brain death is, in one sense, an ethical debate. There is an urgent ethical imperative to formulate, and advocate, the most empirically determinate definition of death. In this respect the brainstem definition was, so to speak, 'chosen on the basis of ethical reflection'.

The brainstem formulation has also been criticized by exponents of other versions of an ontological theory. Green and Wikler (1981) argue that psychological continuity, maintained by continuing higher brain functioning, is necessary for the preservation of personal identity. For Green and Wikler continuous personal identity appears to be the measure of human life. As such, their concept of death is determined by the loss of the capacity for mental activity. Thus: 'if the loss of the capacity for mental activity which occurs at brain death constitutes death, it is not for moral reasons, nor for biological reasons, but for ontological reasons' (ibid:62). On these terms the objective is simply to 'show that the patient ceases to be Jones when brain death strips the body of its psychological traits' (ibid:62).

It must be stressed that there is nothing in this appeal to onto-logical considerations which could invalidate the brainstem formu-lation of death. Those who defend brainstem death would fully agree that the being of Jones has ceased, that Jones has ceased to be, that Jones is no more, when his brain is dead. Insofar as ontology addresses the question of being, then the claim that Jones' being has ceased with the irreversible cessation of his brain-stem, is certainly an ontological one. Moreover, it could never be claimed that Jones' capacity for mental activity has survived the irreversible loss of his brainstem function. Whatever determines the reality of a living being has gone with the cessation of brain-stem function.

It is clear, then, that the brainstem concept of death, which necessarily implies loss of all cognitive functions, is perfectly com-patible with the ontological definition's criteria for personhood. With a dead brainstem there is neither capacity for nor content of consciousness. The point of departure between biological and ontological formulations therefore turns on the status of residual functions when damage is confined to the higher regions leaving most of the brainstem intact.

The difference between the two formulations was astutely sum-marized back in 1979 by A. Earl Walker:

It has been held by some that a person with a complete lack of purposeful responsivity, but still able to breathe and maintain certain spinal or brainstem reflexes, should be con-sidered legally dead. Yet such individuals, who vegetate with-out any sign of recognition or response to the environment, obviously do not have a dead brain. That the degree of functional activity mediated by the brainstem and spinal cord is sufficient for an individual to recognize and to react to the environment is conjectural. Certainly anencephalic monsters, born without any brain substance above the brainstem are able to move about, to carry out certain movements of the

47

arms and legs that appear purposeful, and to react with elaborate motor responses; however, the life such infants possess for a short time is of entirely different quality than that of grown human beings, but the question is unresolved if it is much different from that of a normal neonate.

(Walker, 1979:170)

Detectable differences in the quality of life, as Walker clearly observed, do not even begin to provide grounds for a redefinition of death. This is simply a logical matter: variations in quality of life are manifested as forms of being alive. With continuing brainstem function there can be responses, even if they are not purposeful. The case for biological concepts rests mainly on the maintenance of this clear-cut distinction between the living and the non-living. The objection to ontological or higher brain formulations is further supported, as we shall see, by means of an appeal to slippery slope arguments, or *sorites*, which take at least two forms. The first involves empirical predictions of horrid results in the departure from clear-cut empirical determinants of death; the second, the logical version, refers to the inherent indeterminacy of criteria for ontological definitions.

Numerous criticisms can be made (and have been made) of ontological and higher brain formulations.

The conceptual indeterminacy of personal identity theories

Criteria for personal identity have been extensively discussed by philosophers, theologians, and lay persons, and vary from culture to culture. Arguments in favour of a formulation of death in terms of personal identity often assume an 'essence', the loss of which entails loss of identity. Whether there is such an essence is far from clear and physicians qua physicians would be ill-advised to seek criteria for detecting its loss. Arguments about personal identity are inherently vague and in the recent literature on brain death they have generated questionable distinctions between the death of a person and the death of that person's body, which are meaningless in a clinical context. In many respects the concept of personal identity belongs to a different logical space than concepts relating to life and death and cessation of vital functions. Questions like 'When did Shakespeare die?' and 'When did Shakespeare lose what was essential to his being Shakespeare?' are logically distinct. Shakespeare died when his brain ceased to function but whatever count as the phenomena that gave Shakespeare his personal identity might be radically distinct from the function of his brain.

Personal identity does not have any specific anatomical location. Where is 'me'? Where am 'I' located? When someone says 'Look at me', we usually look at their eyes. But the eyes are not the person. Although a person cannot live without a brain a person is not a brain, for concepts of personal identity can extend to the moral, spiritual, and political status of human beings and an arbitrary selection of other animals and fictional characters. And these concepts need not be tied to psychological functions which occur within the lifespan of the individual.

Personhood is a quality, akin to others like spirit, guts, will, heart, and soul, which are attributed to a being by means of social conventions, not by reference to an individual's physical structure. It is precisely because personhood is bound up with the complex legal and political relationships and attitudes expressed in social life that so little agreement has been reached with regard to when a being can become, or cease to be, a person. Until 1879, when Chief Standing Bear won the right to be recognized as a 'person', North American Indians were not regarded as persons in any legal sense. More recently animal rights supporters have advanced claims of personhood on behalf of dolphins, stressing their brain size and communicative abilities (Daws, 1983:361–71). Among philosophers and theologians there are disagreements as to whether the status of personhood is achieved before birth or much later. Catholic theologians locate the origins of personal identity in conception, whilst some philosophers locate its emergence at a later stage, during infant development. According to Kushner:

> Only gradually in foetal and then infant development does he or she acquire the characteristics of personhood. The process of becoming a person is a lengthy one and even at birth the infant has only some of the necessary psychological attributes such as desires, wants, frustrations and feelings. It will take time for the more complex sets of capacities . . . to develop in the course of interaction between the infant and his environment.
>
> (Kushner, 1984:7)

Central to the appeal to loss of personhood is the argument

49

that there is no significant distinction – as far as the individual is concerned – between brainstem death and the persistent vegetative state in the sense that there is no person there in either case who is capable of meaningful interaction with the environment, nor is there any capacity for having experiences. Puccetti (1988:85), for example, sees two kinds of corpses; those who cannot breathe unaided and a small minority who can.

But suppose it is granted that the individual's life is no longer any use to her; that although her body functions in a vegetative sense, there is no person, no psyche. For the purpose of the argument let it also be assumed that universally agreed criteria for detecting the absence of the psyche have been discovered despite the fact that brainstem function, spontaneous breathing, and heart-beat continue. It might well be argued it is still wrong to treat this as an instance of death, for once determined as dead, steps would have to be taken to prevent the 'corpse' spontaneously breathing by either suffocation, lethal injection, or removal of vital organs. Now, for the purpose of this argument only, let it be assumed that such a course of action would not be harmful to the person – who, so the argument goes, is no longer there. But such invasion of that person's body is still subject to moral criticism out of a sense of respect for an integrated functioning human organism which, despite loss of communicative powers, still commands a different kind of respect from that considered appropriate to a corpse or piece of discarded tissue. It is still the body of that person, and whilst it breathes spontaneously it is subject to the respect due to a member of a moral community.

Moreover, there are well-established grounds for displaying respect towards a being that is fighting death, whether it is deemed to be human or sub-human. Rolston, who argues against the vivisection of comatose patients, reminds us that 'part of the dignity of a living body is revealed in its sustained resistance to death' (Rolston, 1982:337). It might even be argued that despite loss of communicative abilities, a being that is still resisting death retains some token of personal identity which commands respect. On these terms criteria for loss of personal identity would not be fulfilled by patients in persistent vegetative states. Expressions like, 'Jim is hanging on by a thread', can be uttered in contexts where massive, irreversible damage has been inflicted upon the higher brain. That such utterances can convey respect, as well as pity, suggests that it is not uncommon to attribute personhood to

50

beings who have lost all higher brain functions. In this context the wilful destruction of vital processes or removal of organs from a being that is capable of responding to painful stimuli, groaning and gasping for breath, reveals a form of contempt towards our concept of a human being, even if it could ever be established that the psyche had departed.

A slippery slope objection to such practices would be to point out the dangers inherent in a society which exhibited such disregard for the symbolic and moral status of a functioning human body. It might be argued that killing bodies is not as reprehensible as killing people, but killing bodies (if one could ever be sure that only the body was being killed) would be a very large step down a slope on which it might be hard to stop.

There is, however, something absurd in the proposal that one can kill a body but not the person, or that a person can die but not that person's body. One can imagine very bizarre legal proceedings which might turn on the question of whether Smith was killed or his body. Such nonsense is the result of a version of Cartesian dualism which has found its way into the brain death debate.

In a criticism of the Harvard Committee's Report (Ad Hoc Committee, 1968) Hans Jonas detected a version of brain–body dualism in their endorsement of irreversible coma as a concept of death. But Jonas' remarks are more relevant when applied to some of the current personal identity theories.

> I see lurking behind the proposed definition of death, apart from its obvious pragmatic motivation, a curious revenant of the old soul–body dualism. Its new apparition is the dualism of the brain and the body. In a certain analogy to the former it holds that the true human person rests in (or is represented by) the brain, of which the rest of the body is a mere subservient tool. Thus when the brain dies, it is as when the soul departed: what is left are 'mortal remains'. Now nobody will deny that the cerebral aspect is decisive for the human quality of the life of the organism that is man's. The position I advance acknowledges just this by recommending that with the irrecoverable total loss of brain function one should not hold up the naturally ensuing death of the rest of the organism. But it is no less an exaggeration of the cerebral aspect as it was of the conscious soul, to

deny the extracerebral body its share of the identity of the person. The body is uniquely the body of this brain and no other, as the brain is uniquely the brain of this body and no other. What is under the brain's central control, the bodily total, is as individual, as much 'myself', as singular to my identity (fingerprints!), as noninterchangeable, as the controlling (and reciprocally controlled) brain itself. My identity is the identity of the whole organism, even if the higher functions of personhood are seated in the brain. . . . Therefore, the body of the comatose, so long as – even with the help of art – it still breathes, pulses, and functions otherwise, must still be considered a residual continuance of the subject . . . and as such is entitled to some of the sacrosanctity accorded to such a subject by the laws of God and men. That sacrosanctity decrees that it must not be used as a mere means.

(Jonas, 1974:139)

One of the most glaring anomalies in the person-oriented concepts of death is that those who advocate them see no distinction between the absence of responses to the environment in cases involving brainstem death and cases where damage is confined to the higher regions of the brain. Most person-oriented versions simply refer to the absence of experience, lack of consciousness and cognitive abilities. But it is not clear whether this loss of psychic response to the environment has greater significance when determining death than other deprivations. It is simply assumed that interruption of psychic continuity is paramount. But it need not be the case and the least one should expect is some kind of demonstration to justify the priority attributed to psychic functions. One should, for example, expect fairly accurate specifications regarding which reactions to the environment are more significant than others for a diagnosis of death.

The relative importance of psychic continuity is very much determined by culture. Some societies place greater emphasis on psychic continuity than others. Moreover, what counts as loss of psychic continuity is culturally relative. Were psychic continuity elevated into the sole criterion then a physician practising in a typical multi-cultural environment would face almost insurmountable problems in deciding whether to resuscitate or not. But even if it could be determined, with any degree of precision, that personal identity was lost, that 'Jim is no longer with us', this would not provide grounds for a diagnosis of death. It would mean little more than 'Jim is no longer with us in the sense that he is not the Jim we once knew as Jim'. And this state could include a wide range of disorders, both moral and clinical. The loss of a person cannot be equated with the loss of a patient.

The empirical indeterminacy of personal identity theories

Personal identity concepts of death run into difficulties with borderline cases, such as anencephaly or profound dementia. There are much closer similarities between the persistent vegetative state and profound dementia than between the loss of brainstem function and the persistent vegetative state. Moreover, there are clinical objections to a diagnosis of death when there is persisting function in the brainstem. It is still uncertain whether fragments of consciousness or awareness may be mediated by sub-cortical structures. It is particularly difficult to prove that there is total absence of sentience when the brainstem is still functioning. Furthermore, what is meant by the expression 'loss of cognitive faculties'? Does it exclude any type of perception that may, in part, be mediated by the lower part of the brain? If patients in persistent vegetative states are to be considered dead then how much neocortical damage would be necessary for a patient to be labelled vegetative? Their loss of cognitive faculties is usually, but not invariably, irreversible. This potential variation in clinical outcome probably reflects the lack of clinical homogeneity in vegetative patients, and reflects a lack of firm criteria for defining the vegetative state. No physician should diagnose death in such cases (Pallis, 1983).

While death of the brainstem is relatively easy to diagnose, the same cannot be said for death conceived of in terms of the loss of higher functions. 'It is easier to test pupils than to be certain about sentience' (ibid). Diagnosis of the persistent vegetative state may be difficult (Beresford, 1978), and the problem of diagnosing absence of self-awareness should not be underestimated. Exponents of higher brain formulations of death very rarely address the distinction between persistent vegetative states and 'locked in' states, which superficially resemble the former, yet strong evidence suggests awareness and even experience of anguish in these cases (Levy et al., 1987). Unlike clinical tests for brainstem death, which is a once and for all phenomenon, tests for self-awareness may yield differential results. Some patients in persistent vegetative states:

> display a considerable amount of organized behavioural activity in response to sudden or noxious stimuli. Nearly all regain sleep–wake cycles; many display the facial appearance of interest; and some even show emotional fluctuations with occasional infant-like tearing or smiling in response to non-verbal stimuli. ... Others blink constantly to visual threat, startle or close their eyes in response to sudden noises, or demonstrate reflex groping or sucking.
>
> (ibid:679)

Unlike akinetic mutism, where the patient neither moves spontaneously nor in response to stimuli, 'vegetative patients are seldom truly motionless and may even moan' (Dougherty et al., 1981:996). For many physicians, nurses, and relatives, these behavioural manifestations are indicative of the persistence of life and suggest that residual levels of self-awareness cannot be ruled out with certainty.

Several attempts to establish objective laboratory confirmation of absence of self-awareness in patients in persistent vegetative states have involved positron emission tomographic (PET) measurements of regional cerebral blood flow (rCBF) and glucose metabolic rate (rCMR Glc). PET scans of patients in persistent vegetative states have revealed a rCMR Glc reduction of 60 per cent, which is well below the 13 per cent decline reported during non-dreaming sleep in normal persons (Levy et al., 1987). There is also a significant distinction between persistent vegetative states and 'locked-in' states which show a nearer normal level of cerebral metabolism.

At present PET scanning techniques are unlikely to be widely available in UK hospitals. They are expensive, owing to the difficulty in producing radioactive isotopes for the scanners, which at present can only be produced in large particle accelerators known as cyclotrons. However, miniature accelerators are becoming available, and these would reduce costs.

It would seem that PET measurements can provide laboratory confirmation for clinical assessment of certain brain injured patients, especially in the context of distinguishing 'locked-in' states from persistent vegetative states. But whether they amount to objective empirical proof of either death or absence of self-awareness is a philosophical issue that cannot be resolved by appeal to technology. Moreover, whilst the basis of PET measurements may be objective, Levy *et al.* (1987:678) acknowledge that 'different laboratories calculate rCMR Glc and rCBF values in different ways, under different conditions, and for different regions'. And even if cerebral blood flow or glucose metabolic rate measurements provide convincing laboratory evidence of absence of self-awareness, the behavioural aspects of patients in persistent vegetative states are consistent with most intuitions and beliefs concerning life.

Criteria for *irreversible* loss of consciousness require careful definition. Although recovery from persistent vegetative states is extremely rare, anecdotal accounts of dramatic recoveries are very common, if rarely reported in detail. One case which was reported involved:

> a 43-year-old man who remained in a postanoxic vegetative state for 18 months before improving. Although he did not open his eyes or have any motor response to noxious stimuli for 6 months, he then awoke and remained vegetative until a year later, when he spoke and followed commands. After 2 years he scored 100 on the verbal section of the Wechsler Adult Intelligence Scale, but even then three limbs were paralysed and he remained severely disabled.
>
> (Dougherty *et al.*, 1981:997; also Rosenberg *et al.*, 1977:167–8)

Such cases are rare, but they reveal somewhat dramatically the lack of certainty in diagnosing irreversible absence of self-awareness in cases where damage is confined to the higher regions of the brain. Also, even if a suitable definition of absence of consciousness could be found, a determination of the precise time of 'death' in such cases (if one ever accepted that such patients were dead) would be even more difficult. Stanley captured this point precisely when he stated that 'there is, at the present time, no simple operationally sound test for the persistent vegetative state', but that 'there is a certainty about the non-reversibility of brainstem death that does not obtain for decortication' (Stanley, 1987:22).

The respective prognoses of brainstem death and persistent vegetative states are only similar in the initial period. Brainstem death can be determined with absolute precision within at most a few hours, or days. But with the persistent vegetative state the prognosis for non-recovery of cognition or other intellectual functions cannot be determined with any degree of certitude until much later in the course of the patient's illness. After the initial ischemic insult to the brain there is usually a temporary depression of brainstem functions, where the patient may need a ventilator. After a few days, maybe weeks, recovery of the brainstem occurs with a resumption of a normal level of arousal, where ventilation is no longer required. This is often interpreted by relatives as signs of recovery, but frequently it is only an evolution into the persistent vegetative state. Nevertheless a certain diagnosis of the persistent vegetative state involves observations over a considerable length of time. It may take weeks or months before a physician is 'reasonably confident of the severe, irreversible destruction of the cerebral cortex, as judged by the behavioural responses of the patient' (Cranford and Smith, 1979:205).

Diagnosing persistent vegetative states in children is even more problematic. According to one report:

> Several months must elapse after an acute insult in children before a persistent vegetative state can be diagnosed with certainty. In our series eight children examined within one month of the acute illness were in a vegetative state, but when re-examined three to six months after the event three of these children, although still profoundly handicapped, showed varying degrees of awareness and had regained skills.
>
> (Cole *et al.*, 1984)

The ethical implications of indeterminate diagnosis of self-awareness has been outlined by Veatch who has stressed what appear to be insoluble problems in the determination of non-cognitive states. He concludes:

> We must come to grips with the possibility, indeed the probability, that we shall never be able to make precise physiologic measures of the irreversible loss of mental processes. In this case we shall have to follow safer-course policies of using measures to declare death only in cases in which we are convinced that some necessary physical basis for life is missing, even if that means that some dead patients will be treated as alive.
>
> (Veatch, 1978:314)

The inherent indeterminacy of higher brain formulations gives considerable plausibility to slippery slope objections. The significance of such objections is obvious once it is realized that a definition of death based on the loss of higher brain functions can be extended to include a wide range of disorders that should not be considered as death – or even remotely close to death. As Pallis says:

> I am opposed to 'higher brain' formulations of death because they are the first step along a slippery slope. If one starts equating the loss of higher functions with death, then, which higher functions? Damage to one hemisphere or to both? If to one hemisphere, to the verbalising dominant one, or to the 'attentive' non-dominant one? One soon starts arguing frontal versus parietal lobes.
>
> (Pallis, 1983:2)

It might be objected that arguments of this kind involve a mode of fallacious reasoning which illicitly conjoins today's proposed uses with tomorrow's possible abuses. But this objection applies only to some empirical predictions of the slippery slope argument. These may either be sustained or rebutted by further empirical evidence. The ultimate force of the slippery slope argument (which is too often ignored) lies in its exposure of inherent conceptual and clinical uncertainty and ambiguity (Lamb, 1988). It is the inherent indeterminacy of higher brain formulations of death which limits our ability to derive from them adequate clinical criteria or tests.

THE SIGNIFICANCE OF SPONTANEOUS BREATHING

There is no major disagreement between Gervais' ontological formulation of death and the brainstem formulation in the sense that both stress irreversible loss of consciousness. But unlike Gervais, exponents of the brainstem formulation place equal stress on the loss of the capacity to breathe. This is not merely out of conformity with traditional concepts of death, but from an awareness of the problems entailed in defining and locating consciousness. For Gervais, however, human death, as a 'person centred occurrence' is a state of 'permanent unconsciousness' (Gervais, 1987:175) which, according to her thesis, is a characteristic of persistent vegetative states. This, however, is a matter of dispute, but the question we shall examine here is how one deals with a spontaneously breathing corpse. To her credit Gervais meets this problem directly:

> How shall we manage patients who are demonstrably in persistent vegetative states, once we have declared them dead? The status we assign to them, coupled with their retention of spontaneous organismic functioning, present us with an anomaly of the breathing corpse. From an emotional perspective, the situation is pure paradox. Between the declaration of death and preparation for cremation or burial, what should the sequence of actions be? While the removal of feeding tubes will eventually result in organismic cessation, the corpse will meanwhile continue to strain medical resources and care-givers needlessly, and to challenge the sensibilities and well-being of both care-givers and loved ones so long as the organismic shut-down is occurring. From a contractual perspective, some active means of promoting organismic cessation is preferable to the removal of feeding tubes. This active means, to be aesthetically tolerable, must be a simple act with an immediate result – for example, an injection of potassium chloride. Of course, only one who is entirely comfortable with this act should be asked to perform it.
>
> When a patient in a persistent vegetative state is to be an organ donor, the sequence of actions must be different, just as it is now when a brain dead donor is maintained on a respirator until the organ is removed. Neither the passive withdrawal of feeding tubes nor the active injection of potassium chloride would promote the patient's declared interest in being an organ donor – or the recipient's interest in receiving viable organs. Organ removal itself will be the proximate cause of organismic cessation. Again the sensitivities of the medical personnel asked to participate in organ removal must be accommodated.
>
> (ibid:176)

This passage deserves careful consideration. It would seem that a warm, pulsating, spontaneously breathing 'corpse' is only a paradox from an emotional perspective. Presumably, such a perspective is a substandard one which would be abandoned in the light of a more rational approach. This is not the place to examine, in detail, the complex relations between reasons and emotions, or to demonstrate how some emotional reactions have very rational grounds. Of course, many references to emotional perspectives are made in a pejorative way, for example when describing over-reactions, loss of self-control, immature actions, and so on. But the judgement that patients in persistent vegetative states should not be poisoned or dissected for organ transplants is not emotional in the above sense. The perspective here is one that is grounded in long-standing cultural attitudes towards the integrity of the human body, together with sound clinical wisdom. Moreover, if emotional perspectives are suspect, then why should aesthetic perspectives be appealed to when the injection of potassium chloride, or organ removal, is advocated in order to 'promote organismic cessation'? And if such a course is deemed to be in the best 'declared interests' of the patient, as Gervais stresses, then why propose an option for medical personnel to withhold their participation? Surely a course, which is held to be in the patient's best interests and involves risk to no other parties, should be advocated as a fundamental duty of the medical personnel. This reference to the patient's 'declared interest' in organ donation raises an interesting point with regard to policy options for organ procurement. If taken seriously, it implies that the interest should be fulfilled as soon as possible, with the implication that organ donors are entitled to a speedier death than others. Finally, the uncertainty of Gervais' recommendations is merely compounded by the references to the 'strain on medical resources and care-givers'. This issue, though important in the context of treating terminally ill patients, is of no relevance to questions concerning the moment when one ceases to treat a patient and begins to manage a corpse.

ETHICAL CONSIDERATIONS AND HIGHER BRAIN FORMULATIONS

There are three ethical and philosophical positions which have to be addressed when looking at the respective merits of brainstem and higher brain formulations of death and their consequences in terms of organ removal and suspension of therapy. The first is the claim that brainstem death *is* the death of the patient. (This question was answered affirmatively in Chapter 2.) If this is the case then having fulfilled criteria for brainstem death there are no further ethical obligations of the kind which would accrue to a living patient.

The second position is that brainstem death is death of the person but not necessarily the body, which, it is said, may be capable of 'living' with the aid of massive medical intervention. On these terms a diagnosis of brainstem death does not determine death but simply indicates membership of a category of beings 'allowed to die' (Green and Wikler, 1981). This second account was rebutted by Lamb (1985) and is also incompatible with the thesis in Chapter 2 that brainstem death meets all necessary and sufficient grounds for a diagnosis of death.

The third position will be examined here. It rests on the assertion that brainstem death and the persistent vegetative state are, *from an ethical standpoint*, fundamentally similar, and that accordingly there are no ethical objections for both conditions to be classified as dead and thereby equally suitable resources for the procurement of cadaveric organs.

LIFE AND ETHICALLY SIGNIFICANT LIFE

It is sometimes argued that the capacity for moral activity is bound up with the continuance of personal identity, which in turn is dependent upon the physical structures responsible for maintaining cognitive functions. On these terms neither a corpse nor a patient in a persistent vegetative state is capable of initiating morally relevant activity. In reply it should be pointed out that an incapacity to initiate morally significant action, or even respond or be aware of such action, does not provide grounds for the exclusion of any being from membership of a moral community and the entitlement to morally significant attention. Foetuses, corpses, amputated limbs, and even statues, can be accorded morally significant attention. The question of entitlement to morally significant attention has generated much confusion. As a rule the issue is rarely about whether or not a being is entitled to morally significant attention, but rather about which type of morally significant attention is appropriate. A tree or a mountain may be accorded moral significance – even deified – but this carries no imperative to avoid causing it embarrassment.

Nevertheless, considerable support has been expressed for the view that a being deemed incapable of experiencing ethically significant attention is no longer entitled to it. Such a being, so the argument runs, is one lacking the characteristics associated with personal identity where, presumably, personal identity is determined in terms of the structures believed to be responsible for cognition. According to Gillett the 'ability to express and develop' personality

> is crucially dependent upon the intact functioning of his brain (particularly those areas most severely damaged in trauma or anoxia ischemia) which enables him to interact with others and the world around him in a rich and complex manner. Once this crucial enabling condition is removed we are justified in thinking that his body can no longer be seen as the locus of that activity we call the expression of personal identity. If his brain is no longer working and has no prospect of returning to an adequate level of functioning to support this activity, then his liberty as an embodied person has been destroyed.

> (Gillett, 1986:84)

There are two standpoints concerning the appropriate treatment of patients who are deemed to have lost that which makes their lives ethically significant. One standpoint involves advocacy of euthanasia, the other involves appeals to advance the definition of death so as to include persistent vegetative states and other cases where the conditions for ethically significant life are no longer deemed to be present. But whilst there is a clear distinction between criteria for euthanasia and proposed criteria for diagnosing death, there is a sense in which this distinction can lose its significance. If the criteria, in both cases, are based on an appeal to a loss of meaning and capacity to value life – a loss of personhood – then once these criteria are said to have been met it matters little what description is actually given to the set of actions (or for that matter, inactions) which lead to the extinction of remaining vital functions. For in such cases the crucial boundary will have been crossed when a life has been deemed to have lost its meaning.

This risk of blurring the distinction between euthanasia and proposals to redefine death can be seen in two recent contributors to the 'redefinition' debate.

(1) Rachels: Having a life and being alive

According to Rachels there is a sharp distinction between being alive in the biological sense and having a life in a social and moral sense (Rachels, 1986). 'Being alive, in the biological sense', he says, 'is relatively unimportant. One's *life*, by contrast, is immensely important; it is the sum of one's aspirations, decisions, activities, projects and human relationships' (ibid:5). Once one has lost one's life, so to speak, then being alive is of little moral consequence. Rachels' paradigm case is of a woman whose life was being destroyed by Alzheimer's disease. She was killed by her husband as an act of mercy. In such a case, argues Rachels: 'He was not destroying her life; it had already been destroyed by Alzheimer's disease. Thus he was not behaving immorally' (ibid:6).

The question of whether euthanasia in such circumstances is ethically justifiable need not be examined here, for what Rachels' position amounts to, strictly speaking, is the claim that in this case euthanasia did not take place as the woman in question had already 'died' insofar as she had ceased to 'have a life'. What is of importance in the present inquiry is the status of Rachels' distinction between life in the biological sense and life in the social or moral sense, which is presented as if it were simply a matter of presenting alternative concepts and criteria of death for selection. But against this view it must be stressed that criteria meeting the biological concept (brainstem death) is precise and wholly objective; whereas criteria for having a life is indeterminate and subject to social and personal interpretations. Not having a life might well apply to a victim of Alzheimer's disease (although even here there are exceptions, such as the patient so movingly described in Sack's *The Man Who Mistook His Wife For A Hat*). But it might well apply to a wide range of cases, from a putrefying corpse at one extreme to a bored adolescent on the other. Between these two extremes are endless possibilities, including various infirmities associated with age, victims of accidents, the unemployed, the retired, and the majority of the world's population who live on the edge of starvation, lacking the material necessities for having any meaningful life.

(2) Gillett: Alive in an 'ethically interesting' sense

Although Gillett (1986) does not actually propose a redefinition of death to include the persistent vegetative state he comes very close to it when he invokes the expression 'Jim is no longer with us' in the context of describing such cases. Says Gillett:

> When the body of a person has been plunged into a state which will no longer sustain his life as a person we might say, with complete justification, that the soul has departed, no matter what our metaphysical beliefs happen to be.
> ... without 'fiddling about' with the definition of death, we can make the decision that this person is no longer, in an ethically interesting sense, alive. Having made that decision we no longer have in our hands a person who is a patient we must care for but a body in which our former patient has no further interest.
>
> (ibid:85)

Gillett is clearly working within a Cartesian dualistic framework and his ethical cut-off point is when the 'ghost' leaves the machine. However, modern dualists may find the notion of a ghost or incorporeal spirit rather antiquated, so reference is usually made to the loss of certain structures bound up with consciousness. But exactly which structures are specified, and how much loss must be entailed is extremely hard to formulate. Moreover, it is not clear why consciousness should be given such primary ethical significance. Although it has certain connections with ethically significant interactions, such as intentional behaviour and responsibility, this is not the totality of ethical significance. The purely helpless awake in other moral beings a need for respect and nurture. The dead do not possess this capacity. Gillett expresses reservations over the extension of death to include the persistent vegetative state on the grounds that he has not 'pursued the possibilities of a "sorites argument" once this move is made' (ibid:85). But he does indicate that patients in persistent vegetative states could be treated as if they were dead, as they are not alive in 'any ethically interesting sense'.

As we have seen above, the *sorites*, or slippery slope, argument raises fundamental objections against proposals to expand the definition of death to include various non-cognitive states, and the same objections can be applied to proposals to introduce a special category of beings who are as good as dead because they are deemed to be no longer alive in any ethically interesting sense.

No doubt Gillett's arguments are focused on cases involving massive irreversible brain injury where one can say, with reasonable accuracy, that consciousness will never return. But, as we saw earlier, this is an area where imprecision and diagnostic uncertainty prevails. At what point, it may be asked, does Jim pass into that state where he can safely be said to be 'no longer with us'? This judgement is not simply a matter of clinical tests, as in the case of a diagnosis of brainstem death; it involves metaphysical and moral beliefs concerning what it is, or was, to be Jim. To take an extreme view, in a moral context, it may be appropriate to say that 'Jim is still with us' despite the fact that Jim's body was disintegrated in a nuclear explosion. At the other extreme, the judgement that 'Jim is no longer with us' in any ethically interesting sense could be applied to numerous states including moral or religious conversions, depressive withdrawal, dementia, and expulsion/resignation from the Party or the Church. Between these two extremes is a grey area of indeterminacy where clinical observables are weighted according to moral, metaphysical, or religious values.

Criteria meeting a concept of 'no longer alive in any ethically interesting sense' might well be invoked in many social contexts (who would hire a lawyer or an estate agent in such a state?), but one cannot achieve a level of precision and certainty to justify their employment in the context of decisions to authorize suspension of therapy and removal of organs for transplantation purposes.

Apart from slippery slope reservations with proposals to remove various non-cognitive states from the sphere of ethical concern, there are very powerful ethical objections to the practical consequences of a dualistic assumption that psychic features have a greater moral status than the physical aspects of life. In a reply to Gillett, Stanley (1987) poses the crucial question:

Are there really to be no more limits than now obtain for the treatment of cadavers? What if the next of kin wanted to use the kidneys or heart of the body that 'is no longer in any ethically interesting sense alive' for another member of the family who needed a life-saving transplant? Would that decision be justified? What if the next of kin decides that he would like to keep that body (in which the former patient no longer has any interest) 'alive' for as long as technically possible as a living organ bank for possible future family emergencies? Could that decision be justified? Could a death certificate be issued with all of its legal implications, including inheritance of property?

(Stanley, 1987:21)

Stanley's rebuttal here can be identified as an empirical, or 'horrid results' prediction of the end stage of the slippery slope. To extend a definition of death to include decortication (or loss of personhood in this sense) requires that we must 'face squarely a host of implications that seem to run counter to current clinical practice and most current public sentiment, including the implication that all those patients ... in a persistent vegetative state are ethically indistinguishable from cadavers' (ibid:21).

Now the force of the slippery slope appeal to 'horrid results' depends upon there being a degree of consensus regarding the horridness of the end stage. In this example the ethical intuitions of the majority of therapists would indicate a consensus. But what if the very grounds for that consensus is under challenge, as is clear from Gervais' arguments in favour of a redefinition of death? Gervais' strategy is to meet predictions of 'horrid results' with an appeal to a programme of public education that would render those results morally acceptable. The problem here is that such 'educational' programmes can be invoked to justify almost any proposed new boundary, and as a consequence do not provide grounds for accepting the proposals in the first place.

Our current moral intuitions should not be swept aside in favour of appeals which rely on clinical indeterminacy and dubious criteria for personal identity. The notion of a still-breathing corpse is morally repugnant. How, for example, does one dispose of such a being? Should burial or cremation take place whilst respiration continues? Or should someone take responsibility for suffocating the 'corpse' first? And what would be the outcome if a distraught family member suffocated a relative who had been vegetative for months? Would it be homicide? Or would it be seen as unacceptable treatment of a corpse? As Lynn (1983) pointed out when making these criticisms of higher brain formulations, society cannot afford the kind of ambiguity inherent in them. At best higher brain formulations require the advocacy of benign neglect. At worst they imply the advocacy of active euthanasia. Between

65

the two is a slippery slope strewn with conceptual and moral uncertainty. The cognitive and affective components of consciousness may be essential for a meaningful and pleasant life, but they are not necessary and sufficient conditions for a diagnosis of death and authorization of organ removal.

A NOTE ON EUTHANASIA

Although the topic of euthanasia has been raised, arguments in favour of it, or against it, have not been fully addressed here. It has been considered and rejected by the vast majority of medical authorities in the world. If practised by physicians it would make nonsense of their very function as life-savers. All medical research, its equipment, technology, funding, the scientific drive for better drugs and therapies, and greater accuracy, would be called into question. Why do all this when you can terminate a life? This, of course, is not to say that all of scientific medicine's resources should be brought out in full to prolong every life on every occasion by any means. There is simply a need to recognize when to cease efforts to 'treat for living' and when it is ethically necessary, and in the patient's interest, to 'treat for dying' (Kennedy, 1988). That this issue has been confused with discussions about euthanasia, and in particular distinctions between active and passive euthanasia, is an example of philosophical input having little relevance to the technical dilemmas of medical practice. It may be the case that it is useless to apply all the technology available to certain catastrophically brain injured patients whose prognosis is decidedly hopeless. Withdrawing useless forms of therapy whilst maintaining the maximum provision of care and comfort for a recognizable terminal condition is simply 'treating for dying' and should never have been confused with passive euthanasia. This, of course, is not to deny that important ethical issues have to be addressed. But the issue is not whether or not to kill, but when is it in the best interests of a human being to switch from one form of therapy to another?

In one of many pro-euthanasia reports disseminated by the British media the example of voluntary euthanasia, as practised in Holland, was cited in an article published in the *Observer Magazine* as being 'already years ahead of any country in Europe' (Skipworth, 1989:22). The author's belief would appear to be that Holland, where estimates of the annual figure of those who are killed by their physicians vary from 5,000 to 20,000, is somehow more progressive than other countries. This, of course, is a matter of opinion. But where opinion merges with an ill-informed approach to the concept of death then the prospect of serious ethical abuse looms large. This can be seen when the writer of that same article extolling the virtues of Dutch euthanasia refers to the limitations of laws which restrict the practice to voluntary euthanasia. Skipworth cites the case 'of a brain-dead woman who has been kept alive artificially for the past 14 years following an anaesthetist's mistake during a Caesarian operation. Because she had not asked for euthanasia, she cannot receive it' (ibid:22). With such arguments criteria for death are expressed in self-contradictory terms and then muddled with criteria for non-voluntary euthanasia, the morality of which is simply assumed without recourse to reason or justifications.

This is not an isolated case. The record of the media, from the infamous *Panorama* programme broadcast by the BBC in 1981, which presented spurious and sensationalized accounts of survivors of brain death (all of whom were later shown to be not even remote candidates for a diagnosis of brain death), to the steady stream of anti-transplant propaganda, must be seen as a barrier against informed discussion on bioethical issues. To combat such widespread misinformation it is necessary to insist on a well-founded definition of death, and manageable criteria for deciding therapy options for those whose prognosis is fatal. There is no need to court confusion or to gerrymander the definition of death with references to 'not ethically alive' or 'being alive without a life'. It is more accurate to recognize life, but in hopeless conditions treat for dying. If, after all, tests reveal that no improvement in quality of life can be achieved, and a persistent vegetative state has been confirmed, then treatment for dying might be appropriate in that care and comfort are provided until the patient eventually expires naturally without invasive cardio-pulmonary resuscitation and a prolonged period in an ICU. Patients in persistent vegetative states, like dying anencephalic infants, are capable of being loved and pitied in a way that a cadaver is not. While they breathe and live they should not be dissected for organ removal, and requirements for transplant organs should have no influence on decisions regarding their management until brainstem death occurs or is predicted.

CONCLUSION

It is clearly important to define death with some precision in order to know when to stop expensive forms of treatment, in order to keep intensive care facilities available for living patients and in order to seek authorization to procure cadaver organs. To this end the brainstem concept of death has been articulated and defended. But this defence does not require the consideration of cost-benefit factors, or the need for cadaver organs. Such considerations should not be allowed to interfere with judgements concerning the nature or the moment of death.

4

FOETAL TISSUE
TRANSPLANTS

The Gods themselves cannot recall their gifts.
(Alfred, Lord Tennyson, *Tithonus*, 49)

POTENTIAL BENEFITS OF FOETAL
TRANSPLANTATION

Until recently damage to the brain or spinal cord, from injury
or disease, has been considered irreversible. There has been no
satisfactory cure for Parkinson's, or Huntingdon, or Alzheimer's
disease, for paraplegia resulting from spinal cord injury, for
epilepsy, and many other neural tissue injuries. But optimistic
forecasts are being made with regard to these conditions. Animal
experiments have shown that transplants of appropriate foetal
brain tissue to an impaired adult brain can, in some cases, restore
normal function. Taking the process one stage further, human
foetal brain tissue has been used in transplants for patients with
Parkinson's disease in the UK, Cuba, Mexico and Sweden. At
present foetal tissue transplantation is highly experimental and
problems of successful retrieval have not been fully overcome.
There are risks to the recipient which vary according to the kind
of tissue transplanted. Implantation of tissue into recipient brains
is one of the most invasive methods of therapy ever applied.
Nevertheless, in Sweden foetal neural tissue transplants are acceptable, and legal guidelines have been drawn requiring that no whole
brains are grafted; that tissue is only removed from a dead foetus,
and that permission has been given by the woman who consented
to the abortion in the first place. In the UK in 1989 a committee
chaired by the Rev. John Polkinghorne published a *Review of the
Guidance on the Research Use of Foetuses and Foetal Material.*

The committee did not recommend legislation but outlined guidelines which stressed that maternal consent should be obtained before foetal tissue can be used for research or therapy but that consent should not be sought until she has given consent to the termination of the pregnancy. The committee considered it unethical for a woman to conceive in order to produce foetal material for research or transplantation. These proposals were accepted by the British Government. Similar guidelines are under consideration in other countries, although the West German Government has prohibited research on embryos.

Other potential uses of foetal transplants might include foetal pancreatic cells to treat diabetes mellitus (Fine, 1988:5). Experimental evidence suggests that foetal islet cell transplants will restore normal insulin function in diabetes (Robertson, 1988:5). Yet the range of possible applications for foetal cadaver transplants is even wider than is often presented. Myocardial tissue could be obtained from embryos and might be used by cardiologists for the repair of major vessels of the heart. Foetal thymus and liver transplants may also have beneficial effects in the treatment of blood and immune system disorders. Nolan points out that:

> The use of foetal liver cells for treatment of radiation-induced bone marrow failure has been attempted, and these cells may prove helpful for treating other diseases of the bone marrow, such as leukemia and aplastic anaemia, thalassemia and haemophilia. Embryonic and early foetal cells might also be employed in various forms of genetic therapy.
> (Nolan, 1988:13)

Foetal tissue is already in use in the UK to develop vaccines against polio and the rubella virus. One further advantage in using foetal tissue is that it might not be rejected by incompatible recipients as strongly as adult tissue. On the best estimates, the number of patients who could be treated with foetal tissue could possibly reach hundreds of thousands each year.

The most immediate practical application of foetal tissue research is the transplantation of human foetal dopamine-secreting neurons to the brains of patients with Alzheimer's disease and medically unresponsive Parkinson's disease.

It is believed that Alzheimer's disease may be caused partly by the degeneration of cholinergic cells in the part of the brain known as the basal septum. It is the loss of these cells which interrupts

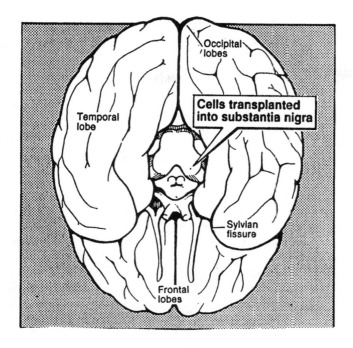

communication between the basal septum and higher parts of the brain, which results in loss of memory and other forms of cognitive impairment. Foetal transplants of young, undeveloped cells into the appropriate parts of the brain would, as they mature, manufacture the substances necessary to restore normal brain function.

Parkinson's disease, however, occurs when neurons degenerate in the region of the substantia nigra. Under normal conditions fibres from these cells secrete dopamine in the forebrain regions which is essential for the regulation of movement. In cases of Parkinsonism, where there is absence of dopamine, the patient suffers from various impairments of motion such as rigidity, difficulty with the initiation of movements and tremor, problems with writing, talking and even swallowing. At present there is no satisfactory cure. Many drugs produce side-effects which can be unacceptable. The disease may also be progressive to the point where normal life is impossible. But animal experiments indicate the possibility of successfully grafting foetal dopaminergic neurons to the brain, thus restoring normal movement. This was originally

71

achieved with rats and monkeys with experimentally induced Parkinson's disease.

Cells from the adrenal medulla (the central part of the adrenal gland) can produce small quantities of dopamine. In 1987 in Mexico City it was announced that a successful operation had taken place involving implanted cells from adrenal glands of Parkinsonian patients into the brains of the same individuals. Since then many teams of neurologists and surgeons have repeated the operation, and at least 100 human Parkinsonian patients have received grafts from adult animal adrenal glands. Adrenal grafts are risky, and there are complications such as hallucinations and depression. Nevertheless, several reports are optimistic, citing post-operative improvements in control of motion, and reduction in drug requirement for the control of the disease (Ferry, 1989:29). Approximately 400 patients around the world have been treated for advanced Parkinson's disease by grafting tissue into their brains. But it has been predicted that 'grafts of foetal dopamine-secreting neurons will be substantially more effective than adrenal grafts' (Fine, 1988:5).

So far over 50 patients have received grafts of human foetal tissue in Sweden, Cuba, the UK, and the US. The results have not been as spectacular as early forecasts indicated, but the attitudes of the brain grafters are optimistic and foetal tissue grafts are being seriously proposed for a wide range of brain damage and diseases, which are presently untreatable (Ferry, 1989:29).

It has been discovered that one of the key factors involved in neuron transplants is that greater success is associated with the age of the donor brain. The most successful are neurons taken from the immature brain, after they have ceased to divide but before they have begun to grow their long fibrous axons. For, if they are taken at later stages of development, the inevitable cutting of these axons during tissue preparation may damage the cells. But if the grafts are taken from much earlier tissue, 'when cells of the brain primordium are still actively dividing, the effect of subsequent transplant growth may resemble that of a brain tumour; moreover the dopamine-secreting cells will be diluted by other irrelevant cell types derived from the same early tissue' (Fine, 1988:5). It so happens that in humans, cell division in the substantia nigra is complete by the eleventh week after conception. Thus the most effective time for transplanting neurons would be between the sixth and twelfth week of foetal development. It is generally agreed that there are no serious immunological obstacles to unrelated foetal neuron transplants.

The arguments in favour of foetal tissue transplants are quite strong. In the UK over 110,000 people suffer from Parkinson's disease. The annual incidence of Parkinson's disease in the USA is 20 per 100,000 of the total population. A similar percentage is found in the UK. No fewer than 60,000 new cases are diagnosed each year (ibid:6). Put this figure against the 150,000 abortions performed each year in the UK, or the 1.3 million voluntarily terminated pregnancies each year in the USA, where (according to 1981 figures) 78 per cent of these were performed between the sixth and eleventh week of gestation (ibid:6), at which time the neural and other tissues are sufficiently well-developed for harvesting and transplantation, and a figure is reached where potential supply of foetal tissue could meet the anticipated demand. Although pancreatic tissue, required in diabetes research, is best when derived from abortions performed between 14 and 16 weeks' gestation, it may still be possible to use tissue retrieved earlier (Robertson, 1988:5).

THE ETHICAL PROBLEMS WITH FOETAL TRANSPLANTS

When considering the ethical problems raised by foetal tissue transplants it is important to restrict discussion to within the boundaries of research proposals. There is little to be gained from considerations of speculative flights of science fiction regarding new forms of life, machine maintained human duplicates, and other teasers for the philosopher's imagination. It must be stressed that current research proposals are strictly related to the removal of tissues from dead foetuses. It is both immoral and illegal to maintain non-viable foetuses ex-utero, or to take tissue from them before they are dead. Current guidelines in the UK stress a limit on the transplantation of foetal fragments such that no 'personality transfer occurs'. This discussion is not even about proposals to interfere with independent human viability. The foetus in question will be dead prior to dissection, as in the case of abortion by suction curettage when the foetus is usually scrambled during its passage through the vacuum cannula. It is the aggregates of cells remaining which are collected for transplantation and research purposes, not a viable foetus.

73

What are the chief ethical objections to foetal tissue research and transplants? There are three closely related objections. First, it is argued that killing and then dissecting a foetus is an abuse to the developing human being. The second objection is that engaging in such practices will brutalize those who perform this work, and the third objection is that it will encourage abortions and even motivate conceptions with the express intention to abort. There is a fourth objection which will be addressed later: that foetal tissue retrieval and transplantation might lead to the sale of foetuses and foetal material, and finally, that demand for foetal material may lead to a situation whereby pregnant women are put at risk. In addition to these objections are ethical problems concerning the authorization of embryo tissue research and trans-plantation.

The first three objections are so closely related that they can be dealt with together. The issue they relate to is the morality of voluntary termination of pregnancy. The morality of elected abortions has been widely discussed in learned journals, the popular media, and various legislative assemblies. Strong views have been expressed and the general standpoints are so familiar that they need not be repeated here. At present, however, voluntary termination of pregnancy, subject to certain conditions, is legally permissible in the USA, the UK, and several other European countries. If the opponents of voluntary termination are correct in stating that it is immoral, then it might be argued that performing an abortion is an abuse to the developing human being, and that those who perform this work are likely to become brutalized, and that any steps likely to increase the number of terminations should be resisted. In short, if voluntary termination is wrong, then so are actions which depend on it, and at least some degree of guilt by association is incurred by those who seek to benefit from the killing of a foetus. Moreover, an assurance that no foetus is ever dissected prior to death would be of no consequence. For on these terms the issue turns on the rightness or wrongness of killing the foetus in the first place.

Nevertheless, the same argument could be applied by those for whom voluntary termination of pregnancy is morally acceptable. If it is right to terminate the life of a foetus then performing a termination is not an act which is likely to brutalize, and further-more, if it is right to do so, then the number of terminations should be irrelevant. If it can be shown that no foetus capable of

74

independent life is killed for research and transplantation, there seems to be no problem. The argument would then turn on the question of whether or not it is right to kill a foetus for the purpose of removal.

On these terms, it would seem that if the arguments against voluntary terminations are persuasive, then the only scope for ethical discussion on foetal tissue transplantation is whether it is morally acceptable to use material from spontaneous abortions. The problem is that material from the latter is less reliable than from voluntary abortions. This is because the possibility of foetal abnormality is too high, and because of various problems concerning the time lag between the actual death of the foetus and its expulsion from the uterus. In any case, most miscarriages occur too early for viable transplantation.

But given the obvious benefits of foetal cadaver research and transplantation, can these virtues be separated from what some people see as the immorality of elected abortion? According to the foregoing discussion the rights and wrongs of abortion and foetal tissue research and transplantation stand or fall together. Yet despite an obvious causal relationship between them, this is not necessarily the case. It could be argued that even if abortion is regarded as wrong, discussions concerning the ethical status of research on embryos and possible transplantation of foetal tissue are an independent issue. The UK Committee, chaired by John Polkinghorne (1989), outlined a 'separation principle' according to which there must be 'a separation of the supply of foetal tissue from its use'. This is to ensure that the need for foetal tissue does not influence decisions to have abortions. One consequence of this principle was the recommendation that whilst informed maternal consent is required for the use of foetal tissue, the woman concerned should have no knowledge of what happens to it.

What is the ethical basis of a separation principle? Robertson (1988), who maintains that the abortion issue and the ethics of foetal research can be treated separately, suggests an analogy with transplant organs taken from homicide victims. If consent is obtained then the victim's organs can be retrieved and distributed to recipients without any suggestion that the surgeon who has received the heart, lung, or kidneys, was an accomplice to murder, even if he or she was aware of the source. By the same token medical students, who use cadavers of murder victims in anatomy, cannot be associated with a crime. Moreover, research on legally obtained cadavers of murder victims cannot, in any way, be said to be responsible for the brutalization of the researchers or contribute to an increase in the homicide rate. 'One may benefit from another's evil act without applauding or approving of that evil', says Robertson (ibid:6).

Against the objections that foetal transplants might encourage women to undergo abortions primarily to produce foetal tissue, it can be replied that among the many reasons why women choose abortions, the desire to produce foetal tissue is likely to remain an insignificant one. And to those who are concerned that the potentially beneficial use of foetal material might legitimize abortions, is the rejoinder that the same fears could have been expressed over the harvesting of organs from homicide victims, and that the need for transplant organs may equally impede proposals to reduce deaths by means of curbs on driving speeds, seat belt legislation, and restrictions on the use of firearms.

If Robertson's analogy between a foetus and an adult cadaver is plausible, then arguments about foetal transplants are independent of the rights and wrongs of abortion. Those who oppose abortion may, however, continue to claim that a wrong has been committed, but need not feel obliged to reject the beneficial consequences of foetal tissue research, provided that the foetus was not conceived and then killed expressly for the production of tissue.

One case has been cited, in this context, which involved the daughter of a man suffering from Alzheimer's disease who asked to be inseminated with her father's sperm so as to provide him with foetal tissue for a neural transplant (Fine, 1988:6). This, indeed, is a problematic grey area. But against this isolated case one must consider the millions of independently motivated terminations when foetal tissue transplants do not raise problems of family members being pressured to conceive and abort to produce foetal tissue. In cases of Parkinson's disease, for example, 'the neural tissue' required 'lacks antigenicity, thus obviating the need for a close match between donor and recipient' (Robertson, 1988:6). Foetal pancreas is, admittedly, more antigenetic, but processing can reduce the importance of a genetic connection (ibid:6).

With regard to the objection that foetal tissue transplantation could encourage a market in foetal material it must be replied that the same objection has been raised in the context of organ transplantation in adult humans. In this respect there is no difference between an adult cadaver and a foetal cadaver. If it is wrong to sell tissues from the former it is equally wrong to sell them from the latter. If it is degrading to treat cadaveric infants and adults as marketable commodities it is degrading to treat cadaveric foetuses in the same way, and it would be equally degrading to pay women to conceive and abort foetal material. Foetuses are not property any more than children are. Although strictly speaking a foetus is not identical to an organ, tumour or discarded tissue, it is, even if unwanted, distinguished by the fact that it possesses a potential to become a member of a moral community; that it possesses a genetic identity, and when dead, though smaller than a human cadaver, it merits a degree of respect. For this reason laws are urgently required to prevent the sale of foetal tissue. In the USA the National Organ Transplant Act of 1984 was amended in 1988 to ban 'sales of foetal organs and subparts thereof' (ibid:10).

It is necessary to consider objections that foetal tissue transplantation may involve unnecessary risks to pregnant women. For example, it has been suggested that it might encourage a tendency to make decisions about the date of termination with the uppermost interest in obtaining viable tissue for transplantation. There is a short answer to this objection: any decision taken with regard to the date of termination, once termination has been authorized, should be taken with reference to the interests of the mother alone. Any other course would be counter to well-established guidelines that the organ provider is entitled to maximum consideration which, as long as she is alive, overrides those of any potential recipient.

One source of objection to foetal tissue research has not yet been considered. This objection concerns the symbolic role of the dead foetus which, in the sense that it is representative of human form, should not be regarded as an experimental object. This objection should, undoubtedly, carry weight against proposals to dissect and research on living foetuses, just as it carries weight against proposals to dissect and perform experiments on live human beings. But given that adult human cadavers can be regarded, under appropriate conditions, as experimental objects for research and anatomical dissection and as sources for the procurement of transplant organs, then there is no essential significance between a dead foetus and any other cadaver in this respect. As a matter of consistency if not respect for the foetus, research on living though non-viable foetuses should not be permitted. This would maintain parity between neonates and foetuses. For similar reasons The National Commission for the Protection of Human Subjects of Biomedical and Behavioural Research (1975), in the USA, rejected proposals to conduct non-therapeutic research on non-viable, or pre-viable, foetuses following separation from the mother. It was held that the non-viability of the foetus should not determine how it was treated and the analogy with dying neonates was maintained. In the UK, a similar report, the Peel Report, arrived at the opposite conclusion, with disturbing consequences if the analogy were extended.

Nevertheless, there are differences between a dead foetus resulting from an elected abortion and a human cadaver, which may be significant in the context of determining who should have the right to authorize the disposal of the foetus for research or transplantation. Should a woman who has decided to abort, under circumstances where it is legally permissible, maintain any rights over the disposal of her foetus?

It might be argued that having decided to terminate her pregnancy, she has foregone any rights concerning the foetal disposal. Harris argues that there is no moral basis for seeking the mother's consent over what happens to an aborted foetus. 'Has she not already abdicated responsibility for the foetus by opting for abortion?' asks Harris (1985:121). Moreover, when the aborted foetus cannot live, or is already dead, Harris sees no moral requirement to seek maternal consent.

> If experimenters ask her for, and are given, permission to experiment on the foetus this permission will not absolve them from the responsibility of deciding for *themselves* whether such a course of action is ethically sound. And if she withholds permission, we must ask what gives her the right to decide that others should not benefit from the research or from transplantation. This would be another case for transplantation orders.
>
> (ibid:122)

Harris is equally dismissive of the view that the mother has quasi property rights by virtue of the fact that the foetus is growing inside her. Deadly and infectious viruses may grow in someone's body without any claim that they are in some way 'owned' by the being who plays host to them. Furthermore, if it were established that a foetus were a person, then prohibitions against slavery would rule out property rights over the foetus (ibid:122).

In contrast Robertson argues that the case for denying the mother's control is not persuasive: 'As a product of her body and potential heir that she has for her own compelling reasons chosen to abort, she may care deeply about whether foetal remains are contributed to research or therapy to help others' (Robertson, 1988:9). Thus, although:

> she cannot insist that foetal remains be used for transplant because no donor has the right to require that intended donees accept anatomical gifts, but she should retain the existing legal right to veto use of foetal remains for transplant research or therapy. Her consent to donation of foetal tissue should be routinely sought.
>
> (ibid:9)

Now the case for giving the woman control, on Robertson's terms, seems to rest on the analogy with organ donation, such as live kidney donation. But this analogy is complicated by the suggestion that, by undergoing voluntary termination for family planning purposes, her interest in the foetus ceases with its removal. In electing an abortion, she is, on these terms, expressing an overriding interest in a premature separation from the foetus, consequently terminating any potential interest which could apply to the foetus. Having fulfilled her primary interest further interest in the foetus would be foregone. If the interest in terminating a life is not maintained as a separate issue from interests in the disposal of the cadaver, then it would seem that Robertson sacrifices the strength of his earlier analogy between the foetus and the adult cadaver, according to which the benefits of retrieving tissue from cadavers are ethically independent of the actions which led to its becoming a cadaver. On these terms it would seem that the mother who has consented to an abortion must forego any directive powers over the disposal of the foetus.

But if the mother is not given directive powers over the foetus, then who should exercise them? One solution is that all foetal tissue removed for family planning purposes should be routinely harvested, when required, for research and transplantation. This would certainly be acceptable in a moral and legal climate where routine harvesting of cadaveric organs takes place. But in the USA, the UK, and some other European countries, where routine organ procurement is not accepted for adult cadavers, the policy of routine harvesting of foetal tissue could well be resisted in order to maintain a degree of consistency between policies concerning foetal cadavers and policies concerning infant and adult cadavers. Nevertheless, routine salvaging of foetal tissue would not only provide more material, it would remove fears that women had been pressured into unwanted pregnancies in order to produce foetal tissue, and pre-empt degrading proposals to undergo pregnancy to sell foetal tissue, and also remove the burden of extra decisions at a difficult time during the contemplation of abortion. It may be that denying a mother direction over the disposal of a dead foetus is the price that has to be paid for maintaining a distinction between the ethics of abortion and embryo transplants.

There are, however, problems concerning the analogy between family consent to donate a cadaver for research and transplantation purposes and the mother's consent to donate an elected foetal cadaver. In the former case the family will not have elected the death of the relative. Now clearly, the aborted foetus cannot be classified as a donor, in the sense that a cadaver could have given prior consent. Moreover, if it were classified as a donor this would presuppose continuity with those who have lived long enough to be regarded as active members of a moral community. And precisely because it is unwanted it cannot be seen as a gift in the way that live kidney donation can be construed. If routine harvesting is beyond consideration, it would appear that any resolution of the problem of authorization must await further clarification regarding the status of the foetus.

Nolan (1988:18), having ruled out maternal consent and routine harvesting of foetal tissue, suggests a compromise whereby 'foetal tissue obtained from ectopic pregnancy' could be collected without setting any dubious ethical precedents. This form of pregnancy involves a life-threatening condition in which the embryo grows outside the uterus, usually in the fallopian tube. Tissue obtained from this source 'is unlikely to have a substantially increased incidence of chromosomal abnormality, may be more likely to encompass a variety of gestational ages, and can be retrieved at the time of surgical intervention' (ibid:18). Since, in most cases, surgical removal is necessary to save the life of the woman, tissues obtained in this context can be offered as gifts (ibid:18). There are, she says, over 75,000 ectopic pregnancies each year; of these a considerable number might be retrieved under conditions where consent could be obtained. These foetuses, argues Nolan, could be seen as gifts, and the analogy with family donors maintained. Like recently deceased infants these foetuses are wanted and are missed. Also, they are not subject to fluctuating social attitudes about abortions and the status of the foetus.

Research on foetal tissue implantation is still at an early and experimental stage, and steps which indicate any move into ethically uncertain areas should not be taken too readily. Nolan's proposal to limit transplantation and research to tissues taken from ectopic pregnancy may not meet the predicted requirements for foetal tissue but it has the merit of not introducing any ethically dubious precedents. Moreover, there are signs that alternatives to the use of foetal tissue may not be that distant. At a conference of the Society for Neuroscience in Toronto in 1988, American and Swedish scientists spoke optimistically of an alternative course for patients suffering from Alzheimer's and Parkinson's disease. This alternative therapy would involve genetically altering tissues taken from the patient, probably skin cells, and grafting them to parts of the brain, thus avoiding the need for 'donor tissue and risks of rejection'. So far this research has been confined to animals but there are optimistic predictions that clinical trials in humans may be less than three years away (Yanchinski, 1988:32). If this turns out to be successful it would be another example of scientific research resolving an ethical problem.

5

ORGAN TRANSPLANTS AND ANENCEPHALIC INFANTS

If society wants to adopt a policy of sacrificing living patients
for their organs it seems very strange – and a very bad
precedent – to start with the most vulnerable patients.

(Capron, 1987:8)

THE BACKGROUND AND ETHICAL ISSUES

The case of baby Gabriel in Canada, 1987, focused attention on
the urgent need to examine the ethical and legal status of proposals
to use anencephalic newborns as organ sources. In the eighth
month of pregnancy ultra sound tests revealed to a Canadian
mother that her foetus suffered from anencephaly. The parents of
the foetus were then faced with three options: induction of labour,
Caesarean section, or carrying the foetus to term in the knowledge
that it could never be a normal infant. They decided to continue
with their plans for natural childbirth but to offer the child's
organs for donation. This plan was executed at the Soldier's Hospital in Orilla, Ontario. Immediately after her birth baby Gabriel
was transferred to the Children's Hospital in Western Ontario.
When she was no longer capable of breathing on her own she
was attached to a ventilator and flown to the transplant site at
Loma Linda University Medical Centre (LLUMC), where prep-
arations were made for organ removal. When death was confirmed
according to criteria for brain death her heart and lungs were
transplanted into a baby boy, Paul. This operation was conducted
within the letter of the law and in accord with guidelines issued
by most countries concerning organ transplantation.

Shortly afterwards, an identical case was reported by Ellen
Goodman in the *International Herald Tribune* on Tuesday 15

82

December 1987, involving a Californian mother who likewise learnt that her foetus was anencephalic. Most of its brain was missing. She was told that it would have no thoughts and no feelings, and that it was doomed to die. It was decided that the baby would be born at Loma Linda. As in the case of baby Gabriel the parents felt that 'something good' could be wrested out of their tragedy. According to a protocol, worked out during 1988, anencephalic infants at LLUMC were ventilated for up to seven days whilst tests were performed to ascertain brain death. In July 1988 LLUMC suspended their protocol, following 13 unsuccessful attempts to obtain organs from such infants, amid criticisms of the consequences for anencephalic infants and fears of the expansion of the categories of potential donors to infants with less severe defects (Shewmon et al., 1989).

There is an urgent requirement for infant organs. In the USA alone between 300 and 450 children with end stage renal disease, 400 to 800 children with liver failure, and 400 to 600 children with complex congenital heart disease, may be helped with transplantation. The precise need for neonatal transplants is not clear in the UK, but one estimate is that about 160 infants are born each year with cardiac malformations of such severity that transplantation would be an appropriate therapeutic choice (Salaman, 1989:622). Although not all anencephalic infants make suitable organ donors, each year between 1,800 and 3,000 babies in the USA are born with anencephaly. There are less anencephalic infant births in the UK because of higher screening programmes, so only about 20 potential anencephalic infants are born each year who may be considered suitable for organ procurement (ibid:622).

Anencephalic infants are considered as valuable sources for organ procurement because, apart from neurological malformation, other organs are regarded as suitable for transplantation. The special status of anencephalic infant organ donors can be appreciated once it is recognized that whilst the majority of adult organ donors are the victims of head injuries very few newborns die in such conditions, a fact which makes it difficult to obtain a sufficient number of organs for infants. And, as transplant techniques continue to improve, demand for infant organs will surely increase. Moreover, demand for infant organs is not limited to potential infant recipients. According to Botkin:

Neonatal kidneys have been successfully used for transplantation in adolescents and adults for a number of years, including kidneys from anencephalic donors. Should these techniques prove feasible for heart and liver transplantation, the demand for neonatal organs may far exceed the supply, even under the most liberal retrieval policies.

(Botkin, 1988:250)

Nevertheless, the number of anencephalic births is declining annually by 5 per cent, and that of live anencephalic births by 2.7 per cent, and further declines are predicted with greater use of prenatal screening (ibid:251). Prenatal alpha-fetoprotein and ultrasonographic screening can now identify all cases of anencephaly with a high degree of certainty (Landwirth, 1988:257).

Given the claims that anencephalic newborns constitute a valuable form of organ source then ethical questions concerning whether this should be done and, if so, how it should be done, must be urgently raised.

Anencephaly (which means literally 'no brain') is generally defined as the congenital absence of skull, scalp and forebrain (cerebral hemispheres). In most cases its cause is unknown but the critical errors in embryogenesis are thought to occur during the first two weeks of gestation. Only 25 to 45 per cent of anencephalics are born alive of whom about 40 per cent survive for 24 hours, although in rare cases anencephalic infants have survived for weeks or months. Only the live births are suitable for organ donation.

Anencephalic infants are not dead according to brainstem or whole brain criteria for death. With brainstem function they can breathe, blink, swallow, react to painful stimuli and possibly suckle. Nevertheless, they do fall into a category of handicapped infants for whom nothing can be done and many believe that great efforts should not be made to prolong their lives. In many hospitals allowing their natural death is routine. This is, of course, quite different from declaring that they are already dead. Many physicians find it both futile and offensive to attempt life-prolonging therapy for anencephalic infants. The US Surgeon-General, Dr C. Everett Koop, who has long resisted voluntary termination of pregnancy and proposals for the accelerated death of handicapped newborns, nevertheless agrees that:

Medicine may *never* have all the solutions to all the problems

84

that occur at birth. I personally foresee no medical solution to a cephalodymus or an anencephalic child. The first is a one-headed twin; the second, a child with virtually no functioning brain at all. In these cases the prognosis is an early and merciful death by natural causes. There are no so-called 'heroic measures' possible and intervention would merely prolong the patient's process of dying. Some of nature's errors are extraordinary and frightening ... but nature also has the kindness to take them away. For such infants, neither medicine nor law can be of any help, and neither medicine nor law should prolong these infants' process of dying.

(Koop, 1982)

Clearly these infants have no hope of benefit but lacking the prospect of benefit is not a sufficient reason for using them as a form of benefit for others. Moreover, hopelessness does not imply that it is morally acceptable to place restrictions on the imperative to provide comfort and relief from suffering. In some cases this imperative might involve removal or withholding certain life-sustaining facilities if it allowed parents to hold and comfort the child during its remaining hours.

Non-voluntary live organ donation is only sanctioned for infants and incompetents (mentally retarded adolescents) who are close family members and then only with regenerating tissues or double organs such as kidneys, and sanctioned with reference to a legal fiction that the living infant donor will have future psychological benefit from the survival of the older relative. As the anencephalic infant is doomed this expedient is irrelevant.

The rather obvious fact that anencephalic infants, strictly speaking, cannot be organ *donors* ought to be stressed. Donation is a gift. Lacking the capacity to give or bequeath they are incapable of becoming donors. Some commentators have recognized this aspect but then express reservations over the use of depersonalizing terms like 'sources', preferring instead the word 'donor' in quotation marks (Fost, 1988). The problem is that quotation marks do not change reality; anencephalic infants are regarded as sources and this is precisely why the issue is ethically controversial.

The policy options for the procurement of organs from anencephalic infants can be distinguished as follows:

85

(1) Maintain cardio-respiratory support until brainstem death occurs.
(2) Redefine brain death in terms of a higher brain formulation, thus allowing anencephalic infants to be diagnosed brain dead and potential sources for organ procurement.
(3) Redefine anencephaly as a special moral and legal category (for example, 'brain absent'), according to which organs can be procured immediately.
(4) Implement a moratorium on anencephalic organ procurement until these proposals have been adequately considered.

Since all of the above-mentioned categories have been strongly advocated by various individuals and institutions concerned with the ethics of organ transplantation it is important to consider the arguments for and against each proposal in turn.

Maintain cardio-respiratory support until the death of the brainstem

According to existing moral and legal guidelines anencephalic infants have legal rights according to their status as persons. As such, removal of organs is illegal whilst they are alive. Their usual mode of death is cardio-respiratory failure which renders them unsuitable for organ retrieval. To maximize successful organ removal under existing guidelines involves the employment of either brainstem or whole brain death criteria which would necessitate putting the infant on a ventilator. Moreover, the maintenance of ventilation for a period prior to and following a diagnosis of death would also be necessary because permitting the infant to cease breathing naturally would result in the impairment of appropriate organs. This intervention creates further problems of its own. In some cases ventilation is likely to prolong the infant's life and may even allow its brainstem to become strong enough to sustain independent breathing for weeks, even months.

Nevertheless, ventilation until brain death was advocated in the Loma Linda protocol for organ prolongation in anencephalic infants (Walters and Ashwal, 1988:20). This protocol relied on the practice of attaching the infant to a ventilator for a maximum of one week while organ quality was ascertained and while waiting for brain death to occur. A Canadian report from the Children's Hospital, Western Ontario (summarized by Annas, 1987:36–8), recommends parental involvement in the form of a prior agreement that the infant will be resuscitated; that periodic testing will be undertaken to determine brain death, including withdrawal of ventilatory support at regular intervals to determine ability to breathe spontaneously; that organ donation is acceptable and that after a definite time limit accepted by the parents – but not more than 14 days – the infant will be removed from the ventilator and allowed to die. There are indications that the lives of these infants are not unduly prolonged by ventilation, although much more research is clearly needed on how anencephalic infants die.

It might be objected that this approach has a limited practicality because it can be difficult to sustain the infant's heartbeat during the observation periods required for the determination of brain death. This has led to proposals to cool the infant prior to death thus preserving the organs until after brain death has been determined. This proposal, however, involves a shift in principle away from the interests of the dying infant. Apart from the problems cooling would create for the diagnosis of brain death, it is likely that the process would be responsible for hastening the infant's death which would, in principle, be not that far removed from killing by dissection.

One argument against the policy of maintaining cardio-respiratory support for the purpose of organ retrieval is that the interest in the infant is strictly determined by an overriding interest in the welfare of the organ recipient, which amounts to the charge that the anencephalic infant is not treated as an end in itself. In reply it can be argued that the therapy employed is not aimed at shortening the life of the potential donor, whose inevitable dying process is simply delayed in order to maintain the viability of salvageable organs. Of course, the therapy is useless from the standpoint of the anencephalic infant, but this seems innocuous so long as there is no breach of the imperative to provide comfort and care for hopelessly incurable conditions. On these terms the management of anencephalic infant donors is not dissimilar to the management of other catastrophically brain injured individuals who are maintained in ICUs in the expectation of brain death and for the sole purpose of organ removal (see Report from the King's Fund Consensus Panel on ICUs, 1989). In such cases, for both the potential adult donor and the anencephalic potential donor the policy is to provide optimal care for the dying patient whilst life can be sustained and then, when further therapy is useless, there is a shift in emphasis from the prolongation of life to the maintenance of organ viability.

It has been objected that there are serious difficulties in diagnosing brain death in anencephalic infants or, for that matter, in infants under seven days of age (Fost, 1988). A working party of the Conference of Medical Royal Colleges and their Faculties in the UK, which was constituted to report on 'Organ Transplantation in Neonates', advised in 1988 that: 'In view of current uncertainties, organs for transplantation should not be removed within the first seven days of life from neonates with beating hearts, even if they satisfy the brainstem criteria which are used in older children and adults.' This caution arose in response to particular difficulties in diagnosing brain death in neonates, especially the risk of errors related to maturation-dependent factors. This may be so. But if brainstem death is accepted as the ultimate mechanism of death then the problem is that of either devising better tests for brain death in these cases or simply waiting until diagnostic certainty is achieved – even if this procedure reduces the provision of viable organs.

Uncertainty over the diagnosis of brain death in neonates led to a moratorium in the UK following the first neonatal cardiac transplant in 1986. Recent guidelines for neonatal transplantation in the UK indicate that 'absence of spontaneous respiration would signify death', a view which is shared by Canadian authorities (Salaman, 1989:623). When formulating guidelines for the determination of death in neonates, and hence criteria for cadaveric organ removal, it is important to maintain a strict analogy with brain death in adults. Despite difficulties in diagnosing infant deaths, as a matter of logic there can only be one form of death. With adults brain death is determined with reference to irreversible apnoea and irreversible loss of consciousness. The same, no less, should apply to infants. In the case of anencephalic infants the absence of forebrain together with irreversible apnoea should meet the requirement for a strict analogy with adult brain death. In this respect it would seem that the guidelines of the UK Working Party of 1988 are satisfactory insofar as they recommend that 'organs for transplantation can be removed from anencephalic infants when two doctors who are not members of the transplant team agree that spontaneous respiration has ceased' (BMA Working Party, 1988). At this point the dead infant may be ventilated for the purpose of organ procurement and the analogy with adult brain dead organ donors maintained.

Against the charge that it is difficult to precisely determine brain death in anencephalic infants it should be stressed that the problems are neither technical nor conceptual – as in the case of determining loss of consciousness or personal identity. As Walters and Ashwal point out: 'No body of data now insists on the determination of brain death in anencephalic infants because the need for determining such data is only recent; lack of data is not due to technical or conceptual difficulties in its collection' (Walters and Ashwal, 1988:24). The same guidelines should apply as are used for other cadaver donors. This involves the assumption, that whilst the recipient may be in a hurry to receive the organs the donor is never in a hurry.

Re-define brain death in terms of higher brain formulations

It has been pointed out that a policy of waiting until brain death has been properly diagnosed and confirmed would inevitably involve a loss of transplantable organs. Under these circumstances why wait until the brainstem ceases to function? Why not harvest the organs earlier? Under present guidelines and legal imperatives such a course is clearly illegal. However, a redefinition of the boundary of brain death in accord with higher brain formulations would mean that anencephalic infants, who lack many of the higher brain structures, although they may possess relatively intact brainstems, could be diagnosed as dead and accordingly organs could be procured without accusations of euthanasia or dissection of the living.

This proposal attempts to avoid any entanglement with euthanasia by acknowledging death before loss of brainstem functions. In its support it has been argued that being beyond conscious life, unable to think or have experience of pain, anencephalic infants do not have any identity as persons. Neurologically speaking they are alive but do not, on Rachels' terms, 'have a life' (Rachels, 1986). Under these circumstances, it is argued, anencephalic infants should be classified under modified brain death guidelines, so as to facilitate organ removal from otherwise hopeless and tragic cases. Thus in 1988 there were proposals to amend the American Uniform Declaration of Death Act, which insists on a diagnosis of 'whole brain death ... including the brainstem', to classify

89

anencephalic infants as dead. It should be stressed that these proposals were not designed to prevent doctors from prolonging
hopeless and unendurable lives, because many anencephalic infants
are routinely allowed to die. The proposals were simply to facilitate organ removal.

Although such proposals are acceptable to proponents of personal identity or ontological definitions of death, who maintain
that death should be determined with reference to the loss or
absence of structures associated with consciousness and cognition,
there are very strong objections.

There is the objection that higher brain formulations are indeterminate and lack diagnostic certainty. Then there are all the objections that have been raised against proposals to equate persistent
vegetative states with death. It is also claimed that the proposed
redefinition is motivated by a need for transplantable organs rather
than respect for the needs of the dying infant. This would simply
confirm the opinions of those who have consistently opposed
brain death definitions on the grounds that they are a charter for
transplant surgeons. To introduce seemingly *ad hoc* redefinitions
of brain death so as to include neonates with viable organs is to
invite doubt over well-established claims regarding the clinical and
theoretical objectivity of brain death.

It might be contended that the motive behind such a redefinition
is morally commendable, namely that it accords with the utilitarian
imperative to maximize the greatest good at the expense only
of those who are incapable of obtaining benefit. Thus from a
utilitarian standpoint the interests of those who will surely die
without transplants overrides those for whom no improvement
can be made. On these terms a redefinition of brain death would
simply facilitate the maximization of the greatest benefit.

The objection to this argument, however, is overwhelming. It
makes the boundary between life and death dependent upon whatever utility is required. It introduces a situation where the interests
of the wider community actually determine the criteria by means
of which a person is deemed to be alive or dead.

Resistance to the proposed amendment to the UDDA eventually
led to its withdrawal. One of the objectors was A.M. Capron,
who warned that:

Adding anencephalics to the category of dead persons would
be a radical change, both in the social and medical under-

90

standing of what it means to be dead and in the social practices surrounding death. Anencephalic infants may be dying, but they are still alive and breathing. Calling them 'dead' will not change basic physiological reality or otherwise cause them to resemble those (cold and nonrespirating) bodies that are appropriate for post-mortem examination and burial.

(Capron, 1987:6)

According to ontological, or personal identity, formulations of death, anencephalic infants are not persons and do not have the capacity to become persons. Caplan (1987) argued that the anencephalic infant can never even develop a 'semblance of personhood', and concluded that the need for organs in other infants outweighs any other considerations. He also pointed out that many parents of anencephalic children would also like to bring something good out of a tragic situation. His proposal was that existing brain death criteria should not apply to anencephalic infants and that there should be less exacting criteria to determine whether they can become organ donors (Caplan, 1987:119–40).

Now this proposal, by running together criteria for death with criteria for organ donation, runs counter to the theoretical requirement for an objective definition of death based solely on the condition of the individual. The situation is even further complicated by the fact that criteria for testing brainstem death are less accurate for very young infants than they are for adults. But this uncertainty does not count for anything in favour of a position demanding loose criteria; rather the implications are that even greater caution should be exercised when diagnosing infant deaths. If there is less certainty in the diagnosis of anencephalic infant deaths then a case could be made for ruling out their use as 'cadaver' donors. This is not merely a question of saving lives through salvaging organs – important and urgent as this is – it is a question of maintaining the objectivity and accuracy of medical diagnosis, without which medicine is a meaningless enterprise. Lack of precision yields an imperative for greater scientific accuracy, which is why the Canadian medical authorities have initiated greater strivings in this area (Annas, 1987:36–8). For ultimately any diagnosis of death must be based on the state and interests of the individual concerned.

It should, however, be acknowledged that therapy given to

anencephalic infants differs from other infants in that they are not normally put on life-support systems for their own interests but solely in the interests of others. In this respect they belong to a 'hopeless' category, where 'hopeless' means no chance of improvement after therapy. However, this category of 'hopeless' also applies to certain victims of massive head injuries who may be admitted to ICUs (yet classified as 'not expected to recover') with a view to harvesting organs *after* a diagnosis of death. In these cases, as with anencephalic infants, there may be an overlap of interests, but a recognition of 'hopelessness' is not a green light to abandon all interest in the existing patient and switch to another's need. Moreover, a 'hopeless' condition does not justify either death *by* organ removal or death *for* organ removal. Such a course would go in the face of all currently held beliefs on the separability of decisions concerning the fate of the potential donor from the needs of the transplant team. Although primarily justified in terms of saving those who will surely die without transplants, at the expense of those soon to die, it would be a regressive step away from the principle of individual care.

A more general objection to the inclusion of anencephalic infants under a redefinition of death can be made on utilitarian grounds. There are good reasons for the prediction that a definition which allows warm, pulsating and respiring beings to be regarded as dead would be counter-productive to the procurement of organs. At least when brainstem death has been determined relatives can be informed and shown how the heaving chest and other apparent vital signs are only functions of the machines, and cease as soon as the bodies are disconnected. Relatives can be truthfully told that switching off the equipment does not cause death, which has already occurred. But any relaxing of the criteria would produce levels of uncertainty such that relatives would never know whether the infant was really dead at the time of organ harvesting.

The appeal to criteria for personhood is of no value to serious discussions concerning therapy options for anencephalic infants and simply exacerbates confusion. Although anencephaly is presented as a paradigm case of loss of personhood by exponents of ontological or higher brain formulations of death (Gervais, 1987; Zaner, 1988), the diversity of views regarding personhood are suggestive of hopeless indeterminacy. Whilst the Catholic Church teaches that all humans are persons from conception onwards some philosophers have drawn the limits of personhood so as to exclude normal newborns (Tooley, 1973), not to mention the vast amount of philosophical literature on disembodied persons.

The insistence that an infant with heartbeat, respiration, and brainstem function is alive is neither immature nor irrational. Bodily function is important in formulating what is meant by life and for some, who do not subscribe to 'higher brain–body' dualism, it may even indicate continuance of personhood. Milunsky points out that:

> Any pediatrician who has examined a live anencephalic newborn will attest to the presence of a heartbeat, respiration and brainstem functions. Indeed, in consoling grief-stricken parents and encouraging them to hold their baby, pediatricians will invariably point to the usually normal other body parts, having first placed a bonnet on the child's head. Pediatricians should not wait to be reminded by commentators such as Capron or Annas that these defective infants are dying but not dead.
>
> (Milunsky, 1988:275)

The foregoing objections to the proposed redefinition of anencephaly in terms of a 'higher brain' formulation of death are neither negative nor conservative. They express an ethical commitment to the value of individual care and entail policy consequences that efforts should be made to improve provisions for care of the dying anencephalic infant whilst, at the same time, taking steps to ensure that such infants can become organ donors *after* a satisfactory diagnosis of brainstem death.

Define anencephaly as a special legal and moral category

One alternative to a redefinition of death in terms of higher brain formulations, which would include spontaneously breathing persistent vegetative states as well as anencephaly, is to define the latter as a special moral and legal category such as 'brain absent' (Harrison, 1986). On these grounds anencephalic infants could be regarded as a potential organ source without violation of current brain death guidelines, and presumably, without accusations of euthanasia.

In a special edition of the *Hastings Center Report* (1988) several contributors drew attention to the claim that pressure for anencephalic organ donation came from the parents of these infants as well as from those requiring organs. Presumably the parents were expressing an altruistic desire to benefit others. It is also argued that removal of organs would not seem to violate any interests of the anencephalic infant whose imminent death is certain. As one of the contributors to the *Hastings Center Report* devoted to this topic asked: 'Who would be opposed to a program that seemed to benefit so many and harm no one?' (Fost, 1988:5). Whilst the principle of autonomy may be invoked to prevent treating anencephalic infants as a means for others, a widened principle of beneficence, it would seem, could be invoked to enable them to benefit others, and their parents.

An initial objection is that it involves a step away from the 'dead donor rule', in that it recognizes a category of living beings who have no interests in keeping their organs. Whilst the arguments in favour are utilitarian, based on the number of possible lives that could be saved, the argument against is deeper and expresses concern over the very meaning of life and death. When facing a situation where one has to choose between saving a life at the expense of losing something abstract like a meaning of life most people would naturally choose to save a life. Real lives are more important than abstract lives. But the issue is not that simple. To save lives it may be necessary to regard some lives as disposable: for example the lives of assailants who are killed as a means to self-defence, or in those horrendous circumstances where starving sailors have been known to draw lots to determine lives which had to be disposed of in the interests of others. But these are extreme circumstances which in no way justify the adoption of an ethical principle which endorses the view that some lives are inherently disposable in the interests of others. One of the reasons is that one can simply go on adding categories of disposable lives as the needs of others increase. Why, in this case, stop with anencephalic infants? One can easily envisage a situation where special categories can be formulated to include victims of Alzheimer's disease, persistent vegetative states and many other neurological disorders who may all become potential non-voluntary organ donors. Moreover, once special categories are introduced, where beings are deemed to have no interest in their organs, why only consider organ transplantation? No doubt someone, somewhere, is working out the potential benefit to mankind of using anencephalic infants for experimental research; they are obviously more suitable than laboratory animals.

It has been argued that organ donation gives a meaning to the anencephalic infant's life. This may be why some parents have indicated approval of organ donation. But as Willke and Andrusko point out, this view is based on a raw utilitarianism which reduces a person to a function, and is a 'profound misreading' of what gives life a meaning, according to which 'the sole utility of a child with a lifespan of a few days becomes organ transplantation' (Willke and Andrusko, 1988:33).

Whilst there is an obvious imperative to respect the wishes of parents of anencephalic infants, arguments which cite parental approval for treating them as a special category of organ donors should be treated with caution. For many it is simply a case of something beneficial being generated out of a tragedy, and this feeling may be very genuine. But the primary interest in an ethic which recognizes respect for life is that of the infant, not the parents, not those awaiting organs, or the wider community. The parents may have good intentions, but society has long departed from the moral tradition that parents may take it upon themselves to decide whether their children should live or die. And the right to kill infants has never been granted to the medical profession. In fact, it is a 'right' which many doctors and nurses would find abhorrent. As Botkin points out: 'the adverse psychological impact of transplant procedures on hospital personnel . . . should not be underestimated, and this would almost certainly be magnified by the use of living infant donors' (Botkin, 1988:253).

The case in favour of designating anencephalic infants as members of a special category has been advanced by The Ethics and Social Impact Committee of the Transplant Policy Center, Ann Arbour, Michigan (1988). The committee rejected proposals to redefine death in terms of permanent loss of consciousness on the grounds that it would be indeterminate and possibly let in other categories. They concluded that provided free consent from the parents was given then anencephalic infants, whose future is radically limited, could become organ sources immediately and not ventilated until brain death criteria were fulfilled. Apart from utilitarian considerations the committee's reasons for endorsing this standpoint were that 'infants born with the top half of their brains missing are so very different from other living infants', and because:

anencephaly is a condition so special, so very different from all others, and one whose diagnosis and prognosis can be established with such manifest certainty, that infants in this most unfortunate condition should be viewed as in a class that is entirely *sui generis*, and for which special rules and laws should apply.

(ibid:28)

The committee also point out that waiting for eventual but inevitable brain death would involve a risk to useful organs. Hence their endorsement of organ transplantation 'without delay'.

Among the merits of this proposal is that it respects the existing definition of death and openly confronts the issue of 'dissection of the living' rather than the endorsement of 'definitional gerrymandering' in order to avoid charges of euthanasia and homicide.

The ethical basis of the committee's proposal is the view that anencephalic infants do not have interests which overrule those possessed by other human beings. Allegedly lacking consciousness, rationality and will, they cannot be regarded as 'ends-in-themselves' and henceforth are not protected by the second form of Kant's categorial imperative, which prohibits using others as means to an end. Hence:

in the case of brain-absent infants, there is no *possibility* of awareness, the physical equipment being totally missing. Thus, in this narrow class of cases, there can be no question about possible human consciousness because it is a physiological impossibility, even during the first few hours before brainstem activity also ceases.

(ibid: 29)

There are, on these grounds, 'no intrinsic interests of anencephalics to be defended' (ibid:29). It would seem that these infants have even fewer interests than laboratory animals since they are deemed to be incapable of experiencing. For example, on the part of the brain-absent donor, 'there are no feelings, no sensitivities, no potentialities, no interests of any kind whatsoever; and therefore, one can be confident that no harm, no pain, no disadvantage of any kind is caused to it' (ibid:29).

Finally, in an anticipation of *sorites* or slippery slope objections that their proposal might open the door to other groups such as microcephalics, hydranencephalics, the comatose and patients in persistent vegetative states, the committee insist on the special uniqueness of anencephaly, stressing that 'anencephalics have an absolutely unique status, and must, in the interests of human decency and beneficence, be treated uniquely' (ibid:29).

Despite the forcefulness and initial attractiveness of the proposal to consider the 'brain-absent' anencephalic infant as a special moral category, there still remain very serious doubts with regard to several of their premises. How unique is anencephaly? Is it easy to diagnose? Can we be absolutely certain that anencephalic infants cannot experience pain and discomfort? Is there absolute proof that even the most rudimentary levels of consciousness are absent? And has the committee satisfactorily rebutted the *sorites* or slippery slope objections, with their claim that anencephaly is a determinate category?

The claim that anencephaly merits a special moral category rests on assumptions concerning the clinical homogeneity of this condition. But although it is easily recognized in most cases, like various non-cognitive states, it manifests itself on a continuum; at one extreme there may be no cerebral tissue at all, and at the other there is rudimentary cerebral function. The brainstem in anencephaly displays a spectrum of involvement from normal to absent. According to most sources diagnosis is fairly obvious and it can be detected quite easily in pregnancy. But not all cases are so straightforward. Unlike the diagnosis of brainstem death, there is no operational definition that includes all cases of anencephaly and excludes everything else (Shewmon, 1988:11). One of the leading textbooks on the subject says that: 'an almost incomprehensible array of synonyms and classifications exists in the literature; many include entities now considered to be pathogenetically unrelated to the anencephaly spectrum' (Lemire, Beckwith, and Warkany, 1978:5).

Anencephaly is sub-divided into two forms:

(i) Holo-anencephaly, which involves complete absence of forebrain and cranium.
(ii) Mero-anencephaly, in which cranium and brain are present in a rudimentary form (Shewmon, 1988:11).

The latter admits of degrees in which the least severe have small skull and scalp defects, forming a continuum with microcephaly, which literally means a small head, although it 'covers a spectrum of problems, including cases in which hemispheres fail to form'

(Capron, 1987:7). Then there is 'holoacrania' and 'meroacrania', which refer to the degree of bone absence, and there are overlaps between anencephaly and another spectrum of congenital malformations called 'encephaloceles', which are described as 'hernias of the brain protruding through a congenital opening of the skull' (Warkany, 1971). In his account of the differential diagnosis of anencephaly Shewmon outlines overlaps between mero-anencephaly, microcephaly and encephalocele, which could be problematic for the classification of anencephaly as a unique condition since the latter 'constitutes a continuous spectrum of its own, at the other end of which are encountered quite functional individuals' (Shewmon, 1988:12).

There are other instances where anencephaly overlaps with other congenital neurological defects. Capron points out that:

> hydranencephalics have normal brain development early in gestation; as a result of some event (such as *in utero* infection) their cerebral hemispheres are destroyed and replaced with fluid. Like anencephalics, hydranencephalics survive depending on the extent to which their brainstems are able to regulate vegetative functioning, but they usually survive somewhat longer because their skulls are intact and thus their brains are not open to infection.
>
> (Capron, 1987:7)

The terms anencephaly, hydranencephaly, and microcephaly refer to distinct clinical conditions, and these differences can be reflected in their respective survival rates and quality of life. Although there are no prospects of improvement in any of these states, and in some of the more extreme cases (though not always) the condition may be lethal, to focus attention solely on non-improvement is to blur fundamental differences and risk stepping into conceptual and clinical indeterminacy. Says Capron: 'Whatever their clinical differences from anencephalic babies, hydranencephalic and some microcephalic infants are *conceptually* indistinguishable if the characteristics separating anencephalics from normal children is their lethal neurological condition' (ibid:7).

Moreover, if these clinical differences are not maintained, if concern is primarily with non-improvement, or as the Ethics and Social Impact Committee put it, a 'future which is so radically limited', then there is a risk of a slippery slope from anencephaly to other neurologically impaired conditions and eventually all dying patients. Already some physicians have expressed an interest in harvesting organs from hydranencephalic infants who usually survive much longer than anencephalic infants, as they 'are actually likely to be *more* attractive sources of organs because of the extra time for development' (quoted by Capron, 1987:7).

It must be stressed, however, that in the vast majority of cases anencephaly is easily diagnosed. But the force of *sorites* or slippery slope objections to the citing of anencephaly as a unique case is bound up with those borderline cases where overlaps may produce diagnostic and conceptual uncertainty. To take the *sorites* argument literally: no one has any problem in recognizing a heap of sand; problems occur when such indeterminacy is built into a complex system of exchange and distribution. Likewise, although anencephaly is, in most cases, easily recognized there are always anomalies involving misdiagnosis in borderline cases. As two contributors to the special *Hastings Center Report* pointed out:

> There is no anomaly that cannot be misdiagnosed, and this holds particularly true for anencephalic infants. For example, one baby entered into LLUMC's protocol was later referred back to an out of state medical center when LLUMC doctors determined the baby was not a true anencephalic.
>
> (Willke and Andrusko, 1988:32)

After citing numerous overlaps between anencephaly and other congenital neurological states, Shewmon acknowledges that in the majority of cases diagnosis is easy. But he warns: 'Nevertheless, the commonly encountered contention that "anencephaly" is so well defined and so distinct from other congenital brain malformations that misdiagnosis cannot occur and that organ harvesting policies limited to "anencephalics" cannot possibly extend to other conditions, is simply false' (Shewmon, 1988:12).

Turning to the questions whether anencephalic infants are capable of experiencing pain and discomfort and whether it can be established that they do not possess even rudimentary levels of consciousness, it is instructive to compare these states with normal infants. Since they share similar neural structures that mediate typical newborn behaviour, anencephalic infants with relatively intact brainstems exhibit many behavioural patterns similar to normal infants, such as: 'purposeless back-and-forth movements

99

of the extremities, sucking and swallowing, normal orofacial expressions to gustatory stimuli, crying, withdrawal from noxious stimuli and wake/sleep cycles' (ibid:13). Whether consciousness and a capacity to suffer exist is a philosophical question which is not answerable by reference to empirical evidence. There is, however, evidence that despite absence of higher brain structures the brainstem is capable of much more complex integrative activity than is usually attributed to it, including some functions generally considered to be 'cortical' (ibid:14). This is considered particularly significant in the newborn. It should also be stressed that the newborn brain does not function like a miniature adult brain; that there is a difference between congenital absence of parts of the infant brain and destruction of parts of an adult's brain, and that the behaviour of decerebrate infants is much closer to that of ordinary newborns than decerebrate adults. This suggests, at least, that one cannot safely assume complete absence of more primitive forms of awareness in anencephalic infants. That is to say, one cannot, with certainty, rule out the possibility of sub-cortical structures taking over certain 'cortical' functions. And as more is learnt about the brainstem function, of its greater complexity than it was hitherto thought of as possessing, there is a need to maintain an open-minded approach to the possibility 'that the subjective experience of anencephalic infants, like their external behaviour, may resemble more those of normal newborns, than of older PVS patients' (ibid:14).

As a check against the rather confident assertion that anencephalic infants, lacking consciousness and a capacity to experience, can be safely regarded as a unique category of fit subjects for immediate organ removal, is Shewmon's warning that 'the inherent uncertainties about infant consciousness are an important yet overlooked factual premise for various ethical analysis' (ibid:14). At the very least anencephalic infants are similar to the laboratory animals – with smaller brains – whom we are obliged to treat humanely.

Is there a need for a moratorium on anencephalic infant organ transplants?

The case in favour of a moratorium is based on the commendable motive that one should not take steps into an ethically uncertain area until the issues have been resolved.

But where does this uncertainty lie? During the past twenty years the case for clear-cut guidelines regarding the determination of brain death have been debated and well established by physicians, philosophers, lawyers and the lay public. During the past decade a similar debate has taken place with regard to the clinical reliability of tests for the brainstem concept of death. Despite the Harvard Committee's reasoning in 1968 that 'obsolete criteria for the definition of death can lead to controversy in obtaining organs for transplantation'; the need for an objective definition of death has been clearly established as a separate issue from the need for transplant organs (Lamb, 1978; 1985). Against this background the plea for a moratorium on anencephalic transplants simply pushes the clock back to a period of uncertainty and confusion between criteria for death and the needs of the transplant team.

ALTERNATIVES

One solution to the moral dilemmas regarding therapy options for anencephalic infants is the removal of the problem, or at least encouraging steps in research and therapy which lead in this direction. Better methods of prognosis through prenatal testing now enable physicians to identify foetuses with prospective serious defects, so that they can be aborted during early pregnancy. In this way developments in prenatal screening would – in all likelihood – reduce the number of anencephalic births. Even with present methods of prenatal diagnosis it is possible to eradicate many disorders like anencephaly and hydranencephaly. According to Shaw:

> Alpha-fetoprotein (AFP) testing can be used as a paradigm for the prevention of neural tube defects (NTD) such as anencephaly, myelomeningocele, spina-bifida, hydrocephalus, and related conditions. All pregnant women could be screened for increased maternal serum (AFP) by a simple and inexpensive test.
>
> (Shaw, 1987:133)

Routine prenatal testing in the UK has already yielded reports of a 60 per cent decline in neural tube defects in some areas (Botkin, 1988:251) and, according to Milunsky, the 'latest data suggests second trimester detection rates of 90 to 100 per cent for anencephaly', such that 'the increasingly smaller number of women not being screened will yield few anencephalic infants ultimately suitable for transplantation' (Milunsky, 1988:275). If those screened and found to be carrying anencephalic infants then underwent selective abortion the number of anencephalic infants would drastically decline, thus eliminating many problems of how to treat anencephalic infants, but leaving the problem of how to increase the supply of infant donor organs unsolved. Shaw estimates that the figure in the USA would drop from 3,000 each year to less than 15 (Shaw, 1987:133).

Under these circumstances many quality of life decisions would be made during routine prenatal care and the burden of severe birth defects would decline. These proposals do not eradicate the moral problems altogether but they do shift the area of decision-making in a way that may cause less anguish. There is less heartbreak attached to decisions to terminate an unsatisfactory pregnancy at the earliest possible moment than is associated with decisions made with regard to severely deformed infants. And given the possibility of dramatically reducing the number of anencephalic births the case in favour of definitional gerrymandering over the concept of death in such cases is weakened. For so little gain it would be unrewarding to renegotiate the definition of death.

CONCLUSION

It thus appears that the anencephalic infant organ donor controversy calls for a serious restatement of the brain death concept. Brain death, or more specifically brainstem death, *is* death, not a convenient set of rules for obtaining organs without raising ethical problems. The objectivity of death is not subject to fluctuations in a potential market for organs. Possessing a functioning brainstem the anencephalic infant is alive and, despite protestations regarding its alleged uniqueness, dissection for organ removal would amount to euthanasia. Problems relating to diagnostic uncertainty with regard to brain death are resolved by either an improvement in the tests, more research, more data, or by simply waiting until certainty is achieved. There is no case for redrafting criteria for brain death, and direct efforts at better methods of preservation techniques that can prevent organs from asphyxial damage are preferable to changes in laws and moral principles regarding dying infants.

The poor quality of an anencephalic infant's life might be cited as evidence against any imperative to keep it alive against all odds. For example, non-treatment of spinal lesions in anencephalic babies is considered acceptable (King, 1987:101). And at least one Roman Catholic moral theologian has recognized that it may be a moral misunderstanding to try to sustain the life of such an infant (McCormick, 1974). The President's Commission have indicated that therapy for anencephalic or cephalodymus infants is 'futile' (President's Commission, 1983:219–20). In a similar vein the BMA's Working Party to Review Guidelines on Euthanasia noted that:

> Any move towards liberalising the active termination of a severely malformed infant's life would herald a serious and incalculable change in the present ethos of medicine. Nevertheless, there are circumstances where the doctor may judge correctly that continuing to treat an infant is cruel and that the doctor should ease the baby's dying rather than prolong it by the intensive use of medical technology.
>
> (BMA Working Party, 1988:1377)

Quite clearly, the problems concerning therapeutic options for anencephalic infants test the very limits of the principle of individual care, and force discussion on what to do in 'hopeless' cases. But given the possibility that, in the long term, prenatal screening might shift the problem to an early stage in foetal development, a fundamental revision of values which forbid harvesting organs from living patients, on which public acceptance of organ transplantation rests, should be resisted. Equations based on the benefits of the many against the inability of a dying infant to benefit are easily weighted in favour of the former. But if accepted they could shift ethical priorities to the point where the benefits of others encroach on the duties to individuals. On these terms the ultimate consequences of proposals to dissect live infants for the benefit of others could undermine the ethical rationale of transplant surgery – its 'do not harm the donor' principle – exacerbate public fears of transplant surgeons as 'organ vultures', and contribute to the gradual exploitation of the vulnerable and the brutalization of society.

6

LIVING DONORS, NON-HUMAN SOURCES, AND CADAVERIC DONORS

Rich gifts wax poor when givers prove unkind.
(Shakespeare, *Hamlet*, III.i,89)

LIVING DONORS

Living organ donors present a problem for the 'do no harm' imperative in medical ethics, as they are said to be harmed by the loss of the relevant organ. This, of course, only affects irreplaceable organs (blood and semen, for instance, are self-replacing and under appropriate conditions can be collected without harm to the donor). There have been various estimates concerning the risks entailed by live organ donation. A 1985 estimate suggested that around twenty donors had died in 'good institutions' throughout the United States after the removal of a single kidney. A University of Minnesota Transplant Center Study in 1974 reported a 28.2 per cent complication rate for live donor nephrectomies (Starzl, 1985:5).

On the other hand, it is widely perceived that if the risk is not too great, an individual who freely wishes to donate an organ should not be prevented from doing so. If there are no undue pressures it is widely agreed that organ donation is one of the finest gestures of fraternity of which human beings are capable. Monsignor Angelini, Bishop of Messine, is reported to have said 'that organ donation ... from a living donor ... is the very highest expression of nobility, in which the Evangelic Commandments of love are concentrated' (Report of the Conference of European Health Ministers, 1987).

The moral issues concerning live donation precede organ transplantation and go back to more ancient discussions on whether persons have a right to mutilate their own bodies. Most of the world's religious codes forbid self-mutilation on the grounds that it is wrong to damage what ultimately belongs to God, or at least over which God alone exercises a final authority. Nevertheless, both religious and secular moral systems permit live transplantation provided they are freely consented to and that donation is not motivated by suicidal or homicidal intentions. No belief system endorses a situation where a recipient benefits as a result of the donor's deliberate death. This being the case, then kidney, bone marrow and corneal transplants, if freely consented to, are morally acceptable.

One objection to live donation involves an appeal to the principle of totality. This is particularly relevant as an argument against donations of live non-regenerating organs. The principle of totality acknowledges that a diseased limb or organ should be amputated or excised for the good of the body as a whole, but it forbids the removal of healthy organs on the grounds that it would threaten the functional integrity of the individual as a whole. On these grounds, so it would seem, the principle rules against live kidney donation.

This objection should not be taken too seriously. Its weakness is revealed once the arbitrariness of the concept of totality is exposed. Humans beings do not exist in a strictly biological sense apart from other humans. A 'total' human being is essentially social, and when removed from a social environment psychological, and possibly physiological, dysfunction can be predicted. As a social being, it can be argued that the principle of totality must include a capacity to co-operate with others, respond to their needs, and receive help. Rationality and morality is also part of this totality, and this implies an awareness of imperatives to come to the help of other beings, and possibly experience some risk, falling short of self-destruction. Given that self-destruction is not an inevitable consequence of kidney donation, it would appear that the risk entailed and modest dysfunction are compatible with the principle of totality, especially when threats to social and psychological totality are apparent, such as the potential loss of a caring and loved relative. It should be clear, also, that the principle of totality can be expanded to cover kidney donations beyond the immediate family, according to the concept of social being that is operative. Many of the world's major religions and political ideologies have long stressed universal duties. Moreover, the principle could be loosely interpreted to include human to animal heterografts if survival of a particular animal was deemed to be essential to the maintenance of the human donor's psychological and social well-being.

There are, however, limits to principles to help others, and in this context it is essential to draw a distinction between what is permissible and what is obligatory. Live organ donation may be justified by drawing attention to the humanitarian desire to benefit others, but this does not justify obligatory harvesting or even undue pressure to donate. An extremely delicate line separates the duty to help others from an obligation to help others. A government mandate of all citizens to donate a pint of blood, or a kidney, would meet a utilitarian requirement for blood and kidneys, but would clearly violate the autonomy of its citizens.

A much-publicized test case on this problem involved a plea for a compulsory bone-marrow transplant, which was sought by a former American asbestos worker, Robert McFall, in 1978. He was told that he had a 25 per cent chance of living without a bone-marrow transplant, but he failed to find a biologically compatible volunteer. McFall brought the suit against his cousin who was believed to be biologically suitable. The cousin refused, expressing a wish that McFall would pull through some other way. The judge denied the transplant request on the grounds that the forcible extraction of bodily tissues 'would defeat the sanctity of the individual' (Varga, 1984:225).

The right not to donate bone marrow, despite an urgent life-saving request, tests the principle of free consent to its limits. The court, in the above ruling, cited in support of its decision the limits of an *actual duty*. But actual duties should be distinguished from what is regarded as a *sense of duty*. One has an actual duty to pay taxes in order, among other things, to contribute to the well-being of others. But certain charitable acts may be performed out of a sense of duty, the extent of which may vary from individual to individual. The law may define the scope of actual duties but morality, which occupies a wider area, exercises its influence regarding the scope of a sense of duty. It is in this latter area that questions concerning the obligations to risk one's own well-being for the well-being of others have to be addressed. There are no abstract blue-prints to solve such problems. Martyrs have sacrificed their lives for the well-being of others, but there are no

106

ethical guidelines which insist on martyrdom. The best guidelines that can be offered concerning a sense of duty would have to refer to the amount of need and the degree of affinity with the person in need. But one thing is clear: decisions bound up with a sense of duty (as opposed to those bound up with actual duties) are exclusively those of the agent concerned; for the beneficiary of such actions may have no intrinsic right to them. In the case of live organ donation, if the decision to donate is exclusively that of the donor, then the strength of the sense of duty may be determined in relation to an awareness of the risks involved considered against the potential benefits that may be bestowed upon the recipient. As bone marrow donation poses little risk to the donor, it would seem that, for a rational moral agent, there is a strong ethical imperative to donate. With kidney donation, where the risk to the donor is greater, then the sense of duty might vary according to predictions of the success or failure of the proposed graft.

Live organ donation has its origins in the 1950s and was usually performed upon identical twins. In 1954 a Massachusetts judge ruled on a pair of identical twins that live kidney donation was acceptable on the grounds that the loss of a brother was worse than the loss of a kidney. At that time tissue rejection was to be expected from all but identical twins. Other donations from family members had to wait until immunosuppressive drugs such as Imuran and Prednisone became available. However, the same reasoning was applied to decisions concerning family donors, even those with no blood relationship, such as husband and wife.

For many years physicians and lay persons have expressed concern over the ethics of live donation. Arguments in favour have stressed the altruistic aspects of live donation whilst opposing arguments have referred to the emotional pressure on family donors. Further questions have been raised with regard to the very nature of voluntary donation. Voluntary donation requires two conditions: freedom from coercion and the volunteer must be competent and have some awareness of the risks and possible consequences. Given the kind of atmosphere in which live donation is required it is not always easy to determine whether the decision is free from psychological pressure, or to adequately assess the volunteer's perception of the risks involved. It is not unusual for families to perceive one family member as less valuable than another. It is not, therefore, unusual to expect pressure on the least valuable to donate a kidney to the more valuable member. On the other hand, in many cases the burden of pressure has been placed on the potential recipient, and many who have received organs from family members have suffered considerable anxiety, including feelings of guilt and a sense of failure if the kidney graft from a brother or sister is rejected.

One justification for the risks entailed in live organ donation from relatives or spouse is that benefit may accrue to the donor, or at least possible benefit may outweigh the risk. In a Massachusetts court a renal transplant was authorized between minors who were twins, despite a rule that a child may not be made the subject of harm unless it was ultimately for its own benefit. The court reasoned that the healthier twin would suffer lasting psychic trauma if he were not allowed to contribute an organ to his brother so that they could enjoy life together. The same reasoning has been applied to kidney transplants involving mentally incompetent 'donors'. Veatch (1978:222–3), in a collection of *Case Studies In Medical Ethics*, refers to an argument in favour of a 17-year-old youth suffering from Down's syndrome donating a kidney to his sister. The case was made out in terms of the youth's own interest since his parents, then aged 63 and 56, would be too old to look after him in the future, whereas his sister could. This is one of several difficult decisions Veatch considers. In most of these cases counselling revealed that the 'incompetent' donor would be likely to suffer psychological damage through not consenting, and that indications of consent had been obtained. But Veatch raises the question, What if the donor had clearly refused consent, despite expert opinion that the child did not understand the decision and would one day regret it? This question remains unanswered. So do questions concerning the agonizing decisions faced by the recipient of the kidney in such conditions.

Live donation from minors and incompetent adults is clearly a highly controversial topic, for it is not always obvious that the principle of free donation has been maintained. This is not guaranteed by the legal device of linking potential benefit with consent. Similar controversies arise in the practice of extracting bone marrow from retarded siblings or minors. When this is done it is justified on the grounds that the risk to the non-consenting 'donor' is minimal. But it still breaches the principle that prohibits the invasion of another person's body without consent. The defence of this practice, that the child or retarded sibling would not object if it understood, is a presumption which scarcely provides a satisfactory basis for ethical conduct in a highly sensitive area.

The problems of live donation may never be fully resolved, but a case can now be made for removing many of them. Proposals to increase the size of the donor pool for bone-marrow, once implemented, should remove many dilemmas concerning the extraction of bone-marrow from relatives. Developments in the technology of organ transplantation, and advances in immunosuppressive therapy, indicate that many agonizing decisions imposed on relatives over live donation can be circumvented. Thus in recent years the practice of procuring kidneys from minors or retarded siblings has declined, as better methods of combating rejection have made it less necessary to rely upon organs obtained from close relatives. Before 1983 cadaver transplants compared unfavourably with intra-family transplants, which had a 30 per cent higher success rate. That year cyclosporin–steroid therapy was introduced, bringing a striking improvement in the prognosis of patients receiving cadaver transplants. By 1985 a one-year cadaveric graft survival rate with cyclosporin was over 75 per cent and sometimes 90 per cent, using unrelated donors (Starzl, 1985:5). Under these more optimistic conditions for cadaveric transplants, physicians, donors, and potential recipients can re-think their policy options. This may well be a case where technology has dissolved an acute ethical dilemma.

Of course at present there is still a shortage of cadaver organs and pressures continue to exist for live donors. In the UK in 1984 the proportion of kidneys from live donors was 12 per cent, and in the USA it was 32 per cent. But the way forward seems clear: greater effort should be made to ensure an adequate supply of cadaver organs, thus gradually phasing out the live donor, and with it the emotional pressures experienced by those concerned.

In practice most countries have allowed the removal of double or regenerative organs from volunteer live donors on the basis of a principle of enlightened consent. As a rule donation of kidneys has been restricted to close genetic relatives. However, it is often recognized that when a potential donor is only a legal relation, such as a spouse, there may be a profound emotional basis for donation. Nevertheless, questions have been raised over the restriction of live donation to family members. Improvements in anti-rejection drugs have made it less important to accept kidneys on the basis of close genetic resemblance. Yet most European countries restrict live donation to relatives. This is presumably out of a genuine concern that any relaxation of regulations on live donation might encourage commercial transactions. Thus in 1987 the Conference of European Health Ministers endorsed the following submission from West Germany:

> Despite the prohibition on fees many people hold the view that the donation from living persons among non-relatives leaves the door open to perverting the intended purpose of transplantations. Even one case of abuse would be sufficient to jeopardize the treatment system of kidney transplantation.
> (Report of the Conference of European Health Ministers, 1987)

The Conference went on to endorse 'a ban on the removal of non-regenerative organs from a living human who is not closely and genetically related to the recipient'. With regard to the transplantation of organs between spouses the Conference simply made a vague reference to 'this sensitive issue' which 'needs to be very carefully considered'.

Now these suggestions reflect confusion and uncertainty. Whilst the Conference endorsed the altruistic aspects of live organ donation, and rightly rejected commercial traffic in organs as a non-altruistic approach, it then placed a limit on the exercise of altruism by restricting live organ donation to family members, and failing even there to make a clear statement about transplants between spouses. This was a clear case of throwing out the baby with the bathwater, where altruistic donation from non-family members was thrown out with proposals for a non-altruistic traffic in organs. But as Evans (1989) points out with reference to current methods of blood donation, a fear of a market in organs is not dealt with by prohibiting donation, but by prohibiting sales. It might also be noted that restricting donations to relatives has not deterred those willing to traffic in organs who falsely present themselves as relatives. Several notorious cases in 1989 came to light when a British hospital was implicated in a scheme whereby Turkish citizens were paid a sum of money in order to donate kidneys in the UK (the *Guardian*, 7 February 1989). Following this incident there were prosecutions in Turkey and legislation to illegalize commercial transactions in organs was introduced by the

UK government, which included a ban on donations from non-relatives.

The case for non-commercial donations from non-relatives deserves a full hearing. Until an adequate supply of cadaveric organs is achieved non-relative donation should be allowed. If it is done for non-commercial reasons and is non-coercive it would display altruism, widen the donor pool, and is could alleviate pressures on relatives to donate.

Wherever live donation is necessary, steps should be taken to ensure that it should be freely decided without pressure. In most countries there are prohibitions against live donation from certain categories or social groups, such as the incompetent or insane, who are deemed unable to make a rational and free decision to donate, or from prisoners who may either feel social pressure to donate or do so in the expectation of reward in the form of custodial relief.

ORGAN REPLACEMENTS
FROM NON-HUMAN SOURCES
Xenografts

Attempts to utilize animal tissue have a long ancestry in medicine, with frequent disastrous results. Shortly after Harvey's discovery of the mechanism of blood circulation came various attempts at animal–human transfusions. The first authenticated transfusion appeared in the mid-1660s. In 1667 Dr Richard Lower conducted a transfusion of lamb's blood into the veins of a 'mildly melancholic man', with no apparent harm (Lamb and Easton, 1984:49). At the same time, the French philosopher, Jean Baptiste Denys, was conducting similar experiments. He was successful with the first three but the fourth patient died. Following trial on a charge of murder his eventual exoneration was accompanied by a decree limiting further transfusions. Denys' description of the results of a transfusion of incompatible blood stands as a warning against letting practical skills run ahead of theoretical knowledge.

> As soon as the blood entered into his Veins, he felt the same heat all along his arm and in the Armpits which he had done before. His Pulse was forthwith raised, and a while after we observed a great Sweat sprinkeled all over his face. His pulse, at this moment was very much altered; and he complained

of a great Pain and Illness in his Stomach and that he should be presently choaked, unless we would let him go . . . By and by he was laid in his bed, and after he had for two hours sustained much violence, vomited up divers liquors which had disturbed his Stomach, he fell into a profound sleep about ten a clock, and slept all that night without intermission till eight a clock the next day . . . When he awakened he seemed wonderfully composed and in his right mind, expressing the Pain and universal weariness he felt in all his members. He pist a large glass full of such black Urine that you would have said it has been mixed with soot.

(Denys, cited by Cohen, 1948:158–9)

Today surgeons use sheep intestine for surgical sutures, cow tendons and bones to replace human ones damaged in accidents, and heart-valves from pigs. And whilst xenografts of bone have a reasonably successful outcome, animal–human transplants of solid organs are, at present, far from successful. In the 1960s there were several chimpanzee–human, baboon–human kidney transplants before widespread dialysis and successful human cadaver kidney transplantation became possible. The first xenograft heart transplant was performed on 21 January 1964 by Dr James D. Hardy in Mississippi, when the heart of a chimpanzee was transplanted into a 68-year-old man who had only about an hour to live, while the potential human donor was still alive (Hardy *et al.*, 1964:1132–39). The chimpanzee's heart functioned for 90 minutes before the patient died. In 1977 a 50-year-old-man lived for three days after receiving a chimpanzee's heart.

The issue of xenograft surgery received maximum publicity in the case of baby Fae, a Californian infant who, in 1984, was kept alive for three weeks after receiving a baboon's heart. The moral issues here involve speciesism, and the ethics of such highly experimental therapy, as there was no prospect of benefit for either the infant or the baboon (Kushner and Belliotti, 1985).

In the wake of the baby Fae experiment there were proposals to establish baboon farms where colonies of primates could be raised to supply hearts for xenografts (ibid). Further proposals are now being considered to put pigs' kidneys into humans and even to breed special pigs as heart donors. Mr John Dark, who runs one of the UK's four heart transplant units, is quoted as saying that he sees 'no ethical problems in breeding pigs and using their hearts. We already use about 1,500 pigs' valves a year in humans with heart valve disease' (the *Guardian*, 6 December 1988). Since 1984 surgeons at Columbia-Presbyterian have been conducting cross-species heart transplants, from monkeys to baboons, and are now prepared to develop a primate-to-human transplant programme (New York Task Force, 1988:25). So far trials indicate that survival rates of primates treated with immunosuppressive drugs are disappointing. Yet considerable funding has been attracted for these projects. In the USA nearly $3.5 million has been pledged to the Columbia-Presbyterian programme, and if the problem of rejection can be mastered, then a new dimension in surgery will have been entered, calling for serious discussion about the status of humans and the higher primates. At present, however, the best one can achieve with a xenograft heart is a time-gaining bridge until a human donor is found. The long-term projections of xenografts are nevertheless more optimistic. If problems of immunological rejection can ever be overcome then the chimpanzee heart might well function as a permanent replacement rather than as a bridge. Advances in genetic engineering techniques could make it possible to introduce human genetic material into pigs which would reduce the chances of rejection.

Apart from the ethical problems regarding the high risk of xenograft surgery there are very serious objections concerning the destruction of sentient creatures for human ends. Chimpanzees, for example, belong to an endangered species. There are about 100,000 left in the world. If they were sought as organ sources their survival would be impossible. Presumably, proposals for chimpanzee organ farms would counter objections based on non-survival. But this raises the question whether it would be right to treat such a complex and highly developed form of life as a source of living spare parts.

Artificial implants

Since earliest times the infirm have resorted to sticks and crutches to get about. Crutches were replaced by wooden legs; wheelchairs and invalid carriages were designed to help those afflicted by various infirmities which restricted mobility; hooks were attached to arms to act as substitutes for severed hands; and further refinements to artificial limbs have accompanied technological developments throughout the centuries. Artificial teeth have been used throughout the history of dentistry, and devices to improve vision can be traced back as far as the Roman Empire. From ear trumpets in the nineteenth century have come sophisticated hearing aids, using computer technology, which also offers a great many devices to aid the handicapped. In the early post-war years there was great enthusiasm for iron lungs, rocking beds and walking braces as a means of restoring to a child with infantile paralysis some meaningful level of life. Arthritic hips, elbows, shoulders, knees, ankles, fingers, toes, as well as penises and breasts, are today routinely replaced by artificial ones. Internal replacements include heart pacemakers, and artificial heart valves made of metal and plastic are frequently implanted. Over 100,000 silicon implants are performed each year. Current research promises spectacular future developments. Work is well under way on artificial eyes for the blind consisting of a small TV capable of transmitting images to a miniature computer that would then send them (through electrodes implanted in the head) to the brain's visual cortex.

Of course many artificial devices are expensive and in short supply. This means waiting lists and selective rationing. The problem of allocating patients to renal dialysis programmes has been an area for ethical concern. But apart from concern over the equitable distribution of artificial organs (which does not touch on issues different from those concerning the allocation of scarce or expensive medical resources) there were no significant philosophical, religious, or moral objections to artificial implants or organ substitutes – until proposals for the artificial heart emerged.

The idea of a totally implantable artificial heart was first mooted in 1964, when the USA National Heart Institute drew up a plan for the construction of a prototype and obtained financial support from Congress for the project. The researchers were unrealistically optimistic for they looked forward to the mass production and implantation of artificial hearts by 1970 (Varga, 1984:236). Despite some limited success with animals, artificial implants into humans did not achieve any significant results. One major problem is the high incidence of strokes and chronic infections, which has not been overcome. The first human implantation of an artificial heart was performed in Texas in 1969 on a dying patient, Haskelle Karp, who survived for a further 65 hours with it before receiving a human heart. He died shortly after. In 1977 a woman in Zurich survived for two days with an artificial heart (ibid:23–7). The initial belief that an artificial heart might function as a permanent replacement has given way to more realistic therapy. Artificial hearts are presently used, in a limited sense, as 'bridges' to assist survival until a donor becomes available. As of January 1987, some 17 US transplant centres were using artificial heart 'bridges', and 63 patients had been implanted with such a device (New York Task Force, 1988:18). The number of artificial hearts and ventricular assistance devices currently functioning as bridges is 200 world-wide (Gil, 1989:24).

The deeper ethical and philosophical aspects of artificial heart implants surfaced in the widely discussed case of Dr Barney Clark, a retired American dentist who received an artificial heart in 1982. Dr Clark's own defective heart was replaced with a device made of polyurethane. The motor driving the heart was too large to be implanted so it was placed in a cart which the patient had to push around. He lived for 112 days, and his death was caused by the failure of most of his other organs, but not by the failure of the heart, which went on pumping blood to a mass of dead organs, thus demonstrating the separability of the heart function from the mechanism of death. The longest survivor with an artificial heart was William Schroeder, who lived for 620 days, but during that time he suffered four strokes and developed chronic infections which sapped his strength (ibid:24).

The suffering endured by Barney Clark and William Schroeder and their families certainly raises ethical problems concerning the extent to which doctors should strive to maintain life. But this limited success may bring hope for the future; hope that an artificial heart is not an impossible dream, and that with sufficient technological improvements artificial implants could reduce waiting lists for human organs.

There are, however, several problems with artificial hearts which ethicists ought to address. It is frequently objected that because the costs are enormous, resources should be redirected to where they will maximize benefit. There is no satisfactory answer to this objection, for it could be applied to any branch of medical or scientific research. This objection has been raised against kidney dialysis, cardiac transplants, and many other forms of expensive therapy. Perhaps the best defence of proposals for expensive research and therapy are plausible predictions concerning future cost-reductions (with mass-production) and assurances of potential benefits.

There are also psychological problems associated with the symbolic role of the heart in Western culture. But these are no more significant than those associated with human cadaver heart transplants. If it were possible for a satisfactory quality of life to be ensured with an artificial heart, any associated psychological problems could be resolved by means of psychiatric counselling.

Nevertheless, the potential for an artificial heart, as in the case of Barney Clark, to go on pumping after the death of most of the patient's tissues has raised problems concerning the definition of death. According to Varga:

> The mechanical pump replacing a heart can function for a great number of years. It may keep pumping even at an age when other organs have deteriorated. Should the artificial heart be stopped the way one turns off the motor of a car when one arrives at a destination? Who would do it? What principles would be used to determine that a person has lived long enough or has already arrived at the end of his earthly pilgrimage and that the motor of the artificial heart should be stopped?
>
> (Varga, 1984:239)

These questions, however, assume that the appropriate concept of death is the traditional cardio-respiratory one. On these terms the decision to turn off the motor which drives the pump is presented as a dilemma concerning the termination of life. But the adoption of brainstem or whole brain criteria for death (which stresses the separability of death from cessation of cardio-respiratory function) will resolve these problems, as it has with human cadaver transplants. Whereas permanent loss of heartbeat can readily be seen as an obvious indicator of brainstem death, it is not death itself. But once brainstem death has been determined on neurological grounds, then the functions of the mechanical heart have no more significance than any other artifacts employed to maintain functions in individual organs.

In recent years highly controversial proposals have been involved in research on a nuclear powered heart, which was abandoned in the light of serious ethical objections. Around 250 grams of plutonium 238 in a sealed capsule in the thoracic cavity could produce enough energy for more than a lifetime. There is, of course, a distinct possibility of a lethal blood disease within ten years, but this prospect is better than immediate death through heart failure. The overriding objection, however, was the threat that such a walking source of time-bomb would pose to others. Can radiation be sufficiently suppressed so that others are not harmed? A person with a nuclear heart might be involved in an accident, the device being crushed and releasing radio-active material. One issue of concern was that 'terrorists might kidnap and kill a number of persons with plutonium-fuelled hearts and get enough material for a atom bomb' (ibid:240). Of course it could be replied that these risks already exist with the transport of plutonium for military and industrial projects. The question is really whether society is prepared to accept any further increase in the risks.

A major solution to ethical problems posed by animal-to-human and live inter-human donations is to be found in a programme for the development of artificial organs. There are admittedly tremendous difficulties. The artificial heart is at present impracticable and an artificial liver is beyond human capacity. But notwithstanding these difficulties a guiding principle on organ replacement should be to investigate very carefully any proposals that would inhibit such research. In this context proposals for a market in organ sales should be strongly resisted lest they encourage the vested interests of organ suppliers and brokers, who may use all the power at their disposal to discourage alternatives to their lucrative trade.

CADAVER DONORS

The most suitable cadaveric donors are brainstem dead individuals who have died in ICUs, who are younger than 35 (40 for women), and who have no history of organic heart disease. Improvements in techniques of preserving and transporting cadaveric organs have emphasized how greatly the dead can contribute to the well-being of the living. In 1978 the introduction of safe hypothermic preservation of donor hearts for periods of up to seven hours dramatically enlarged the pool of donor organs and facilitated the transport of cadaveric hearts. In the USA there are between 17,000 and 26,000 diagnoses of brain death each year. In the UK the estimated figure is 4,000.

Guidelines in most transplant centres stress that up to the time of death, every effort should be maintained to save the potential donor's life, including emergency treatment of injuries, maintenance of blood-pressure, blood transfusions, and other appropriate therapy. By the time the transplant surgeon appears on the scene the decision has already been made to switch off the ventilator, brainstem death having been ascertained. Only when brainstem death has been confirmed does a shift in priorities occur (from prolongation of life to the maintenance of organ viability).

In 1968 the Harvard Report made two important recommendations:

(i) that a declaration of death should be made before ventilatory withdrawal, and
(ii) that the physicians responsible for declaring death and switching off the ventilator should not be connected with any intended transplantation procedures (Harvard Report, 1968).

In 1969 a UK Advisory Group on transplantation problems (McLennan Report, 1969) drew attention to the need to separate the management of seriously ill patients from considerations of organ donation, stressing that the doctor responsible for the care of the potential donor should not be the doctor responsible for the potential recipient. In addition, it is incumbent upon UK transplant surgeons, under the Human Tissue Act 1961, to satisfy themselves that the donor's death has occurred.

In the interests of both scientific accuracy and ethical propriety it is essential to separate questions related to the need to obtain organs for transplantation from questions related to the conceptual and factual aspects of ascertaining death. There is a great demand for more donors, and this will certainly grow. Under these circumstances physicians can be subjected to conflicting moral pressures when the organs of one patient can be used to save the life of another. To avoid potential conflicts between the attending physician and the requirements of the transplant team, practices have been consolidated which ensure that the donor's physician should have no role in the transplantation procedure itself. For this reason the Judicial Council of the American Medical Association requires that the donor's death be determined by someone other than the recipient's physician. Similarly the Committee on Morals and Ethics of the Transplantation Society of the USA says that 'acceptance of death should be made and declared by at least two physicians whose primary responsibility is care of the potential donor and is independent of the transplant team'. The same situation pertains in the UK.

The motive behind these requirements to separate those responsible for the diagnosis of death from those concerned with transplantation procedures was to ensure that the need for organs never interfered with the objective judgement that the patient was dead. A clearly defined concept of death (and appropriate criteria for diagnosing death on neurological grounds) would help procure cadaver organs in optimal condition for transplantation. But it is essential that statutes or guidelines on brainstem death should avoid the serious risk of running together criteria for diagnosing brain death with legislation and/or guidelines for the removal of organs. In 1976 the European Committee on Legal Co-operation fell into precisely this trap. It underwrote the following positions:

(1) It should be possible for the removal of cadaver organs to be effected from the moment when it was established that the donor had irreversibly lost all his cerebral functions even though the function of other organs might have been preserved.

(2) Legislation should move towards the adoption of presumed consent for the removal of cadaver organs if circumstances give reason to believe that the family of the donor do not or would not have objected.

(cited by Walton 1980:13)

These two statements illicitly conjoin proposals for brain-related criteria of death and legislation permitting the removal of cadaveric organs. The proposals are then linked with a further proposal to shift the burden for permission to remove cadaveric organs.

In the 1970s several American states adopted brain death statutes, some of which were attached to the Anatomical Gift Act. Capron's account of a situation which arose out of Connecticut's attempt to link criteria for brain death with organ donation reveals the scope for legal confusion which this kind of statute created. The case involved:

a young woman who had lost all brain functioning as a result of general anaesthesia during dental surgery. She was not a potential organ donor, however, and the court held that she was therefore not dead – although she could have been so declared had she been a potential donor. Only when the public prosecutor reversed his original stand – for this one case – and agreed not to bring charges, did the physician

119

feel he could follow through on his medical diagnosis of death and cease artificial support.

(Capron, 1988:164)

Confusion of this sort stems from earlier attempts to come to terms with the phenomenon of brain death. In many countries statutes and guidelines concerning the diagnosis of brain death have been presented in terms which suggest that the objective was the procurement of organs. In the 1960s early attempts to define brain death were presented in terms of factors extraneous to the patient's welfare. The Harvard Report (1968) itself, for example, gave two practical reasons for a definition of death:

(1) Relief of the patient, kin, and medical resources from the burden of indefinitely prolonged coma.
(2) Removal of controversy with regard to the obtaining of organs for transplantation.

There is nothing objectionable in these proposals in so far as the primary rationale behind the redefinition of death was to enable a physician to terminate treatment when there was no longer a patient to treat. There is, clearly, an ethical imperative to reduce the period of anxiety for relatives. There have been cases of relatives paying over $2,000 a day to keep a corpse ventilated (President's Commission, 1981:24). But objections to the second reason adduced in the Harvard Report were raised by Hans Jonas, who argued that freedom for organ use is not covered by the primary rationale; that is, the interest of the patient. Jonas stressed that the theoretical requirement to define death is one thing (and an essential thing if the patient's interests are uppermost) but that the requirement for organ transplants (even to save lives) is the intrusion into the situation of another interest. Commenting on the Harvard Report, Jonas said:

> I contend that pure as this interest (viz., to save lives) is in itself, its intrusion into the *theoretical* attempt to define death makes the attempt impure; the Harvard Committee should never have allowed itself to adulterate the purity of its scientific case by baiting it with the prospect of this *extraneous* though extremely appealing gain.
>
> (Jonas 1974:133)

Jonas's concern was not with theoretical purity for its own sake.

120

He was rightly worried about the policy consequences of this impurity, once a need for the harvesting of organs is built into the definition of death. Stories about 'human vegetables' lingering on for months (while their organs could be used to save other lives) must never be allowed to influence criteria for determining death. Wherever such arguments are raised they must be seen as advocacy for euthanasia or dissection of the living, and their pros and cons evaluated in this light. The fact that other humans might benefit from organs obtained from patients in vegetative states is no reason for the assimilation of these states with death. *Discussions regarding the worth of a life should never replace discussions about the existence of a life.* The term 'vegetative state' refers to the clinical condition of a living being; there is no way in which it can be seen as anything other than an instance of life.

To avoid the need for transplant organs interfering with decisions concerning the diagnosis of death some countries have proposed tougher guidelines for a determination of death when transplantation is under consideration. In several European countries there are legal requirements which specify that a whole team of doctors must agree over the diagnosis of death in the case of a potential donor. Some countries have proposed what are believed to be more stringent tests for potential brain dead organ donors. The Report of the Swedish Committee on Defining Death (1984) recommended angiographic tests whenever transplantation is envisaged, and also recommended that the Swedish Transplant Act should allow potential donors to issue prohibitions (binding on both next of kin and medical personnel) against the removal of organs 'prior to the discontinuation of circulatory support'. This latter recommendation, as one critic pointed out, subverts 'the main purpose of the report – namely to convince people that the brain dead are truly dead' (Pallis, 1985:666).

The reason for these extra provisions for diagnosing brain death in potential organ donors is, no doubt, to allay public fears of a premature diagnosis of death for the purpose of organ procurement. But it is questionable whether these requirements reduce public suspicions as much as they create them. They certainly introduce an absurd suggestion that there is a special kind of death for organ donors, and perpetuate mistaken beliefs that diagnosing brain death is a hit or miss affair lacking precision. As a matter of consistency, at least, criteria for diagnosing the deaths of organ donors should be exactly the same as for those for whom immediate burial or cremation is intended. The current UK practice of requesting agreement from two consultants over a diagnosis of brain death – whether or not transplantation is intended – is quite adequate. Despite the good intentions behind proposals to assure the public that the objectives of the transplant team should not encroach upon the treatment available to the potential donor there is no need for more stringent criteria in such cases.

The requirement for objective criteria for death and hence cessation of therapy must be shown to be independent of any external requirements. If organ transplantation had never developed, or if it were prohibited, it would be necessary to seek reliable criteria to ascertain death. Criteria for death based on a requirement for transplantable organs is both scientifically and morally unacceptable. As the Report of the Conference of European Health Ministers (1987) noted: 'it would be preferable by far for man's future survival to have to abandon transplantation than to agree to remove vital organs from individuals who are not really dead.'

CULTURAL VALUES AND TRANSPLANTS

Respect for the body of the deceased is a feature of all religious belief systems and secular moral codes. The body represents the past memory of life which should be kept as close as possible to the image of the loved one. For this reason the idea of mutilation of the body is unacceptable. Although a cadaver is not a person it deserves respect because it was that person's body. To lose respect for the body of a dead human being would mean disrespect for that person, the next of kin, and ultimately for human beings in general.

Although respect for the deceased takes different forms in different cultures, for the most part violation of the body's integrity for therapeutic purposes, such as organ transplantation, is not regarded as disrespect. At least no Western Church has adopted an unfavourable stance towards organ removal. Jewish, Christian, and Buddhist countries, despite prohibitions on the mutilation of corpses, permit cadaveric transplants provided prior consent of the deceased – or family consent – has been obtained.

The respect accorded to dead bodies in the Muslim faith rules out the study of anatomy on indigenous corpses. Post-mortems are rare in Islamic countries. But in 1982 organ donation after death was declared halal (permissible) by the Senior 'Ulama'

Commission, the highest religious authority in such matters, in Saudi Arabia. According to Islamic teachings a man is answerable to Allah for the good or bad use made of his organs during his life-time. If he makes a will donating his organs for saving other lives he is eligible for reward in the hereafter. If, as one Islamic expert points out, 'In Islam respect for the living is greater than respect for the dead,' then cadaveric transplantation to save lives is acceptable (Moulavi, M.H. Babu Sahib, 1984).

Nevertheless, there are sources of resistance to organ transplantation which deserve consideration. An important aspect of resistance to routine harvesting of cadaveric organs is the symbolic role which is assigned to the dead body. This role should not be underestimated, even though the interests of the living may outweigh those of the dead. Joel Feinberg (1985) cites a case which brings out the importance of such symbolism. In 1978 the Department of Transport in the USA contracted with several university laboratories to test designs for automobiles in actual crashes at varying velocities. Dummies had proven unsatisfactory. Some researchers – with the consent of the relatives – had substituted human cadavers. After a public outcry the tests were stopped, despite the Department of Transport's protest that such a decision would set back progress on safety protection for years. The grounds for the prohibition of these tests were that 'the use of human cadavers for vehicle safety research violated fundamental notions of morality and human dignity' (cited by Feinberg, 1985:31).

It should be stressed that no coercive measures were employed. Research workers were not coerced and the tests were conducted in private. Relatives had expressed consent and prior consent to donation for experimental purposes had been indicated by the deceased. What then, is the difference between this project, designed to save lives, and the use of cadavers for laboratory or transplantation purposes?

The only difference is the violent 'assault' on the cadavers during the car crashes. But the violence was not experienced violence. No pain or discomfort could possibly have been inflicted upon the 'victims'. The issue at stake appears to concern the symbolic role of the human cadaver. Violent assault on a cadaver is an assault on the important symbolic role assigned to the newly dead.

According to Feinberg symbolic fears of this kind, though

culturally significant, should not outweigh the imperative to save lives. Certainly objections to the routine salvaging of cadaveric organs based on symbolic fears should not impede research to improve life-expectancy. To drive home this point Feinberg draws an analogy with William James' story of a Russian aristocrat who wept over a fictional tragedy in a theatre while her coachman froze to death outside in her carriage. In such cases the symbolic has outweighed the real.

There is merit in Feinberg's argument. But in reply it must be stressed that symbols are important to the very fabric of society. A society with no symbolic values for the dead is little short of savagery. Moreover, a body is not just a symbol. The newly dead continue as a presence, which is why they are referred to as deceased. The absence of the life that once existed has a very real presence. This aspect can be seen in Leon Kass's account of his experience of the sudden death of a close friend, a man who once possessed considerable intelligence and personality.

> I walked briskly to the hospital room where I had visited him during several previous hospitalizations. I asked the nurse who was leaving his room, how he was doing. 'Don't you know?' she replied, 'Mr — expired an hour ago.' I entered the room thunderstruck. There he lay, peacefully, a frail figure in a large bed, half-smiling, as if in a pleasant dream. Dreaming I would have thought had I not met the nurse. Moments later I found myself on my knees at the foot of the bed, full of awe and horror. Over and over I asked myself, 'Where is he? Where did he go? Where is the mind, that learning and understanding, those unwritten books, that no-one will now write?' There he lay, or seemed to lay, but lay not; there he was or seemed to be, but was not. The body, the still warm and undisfigured body, identical in looks to what I had seen the day before, mocked me with its unintentional dissembling and camouflage of extinction. Here there was vastly less than meets the eye. The dead body may be more than what our science teaches, but it is also less than what it appears to us to be. The body may be more than stuff, but the man seems more than the body.
>
> (Kass, 1985:21)

Kass's reaction here is neither pure sentiment nor can he be

124

accused of taking the symbol too far. Awe, horror, sense of both presence and loss, are important to the identity of human beings. A corpse is no longer a man or a woman, but its recognizable form in death still retains an identity; it is no longer the person that was, but it compels us to think of the being who was once inseparable from it. The expression 'George died yesterday and he will be buried tomorrow' stresses this continuity between life and death. This way of speaking, which indicates a continuity between George alive and George dead (although he cannot be the subject of anything after his death) contrast sharply with a strict application of an analytic reductionism that sees error in the sense that if George died yesterday he cannot be the subject of any activities in the future.

The foregoing discussion should not be taken as a knockdown argument against the harvesting of cadaveric organs. It simply draws attention to the fact that other moral considerations than those presented in most utilitarian arguments have force and should be respected. These considerations may not, in the end, overrule the imperative to secure viable organs for the living. But they should count heavily on the side of those (be they patients or their relatives and loved ones) who prefer not to donate.

7

POLICIES FOR ALLOCATING AND PROCURING ORGANS

Am I my brother's keeper?

(Genesis, 4:9)

SHORTAGE OF ORGANS

Organ transplantation has given hope when formerly death was inevitable. But the replacement of vital organs is not merely giving the hope of extended life to those who would otherwise die. The era of transplantation highlights major moral problems in medicine concerning the very role of physicians, patient autonomy, and respect for the dying and the dead. It also focuses attention on one of the permanent problems of medicine – the allocation of resources. This problem has always existed, and has been handled in various ways from privatized medicine to charity-run medical provisions and the UK National Health Service. But with the development of vital organ transplants, human body parts such as hearts, lungs, kidneys and livers have become a paradigm of scarce resources.

An indication of the scale of organ transplantations in Europe can be seen by noting that in 1984 the total number of renal transplants was 7,700, but by the end of January 1985, the number that year had already reached 2,454. Refinements in systems for tissue and blood typing have contributed to a rapid decline in the risk of transplants being rejected. This, together with the development of immunosuppressive drugs, is particularly applicable with regard to renal transplantation and has facilitated the use of genetically non-identical cadaveric donors on a large scale. Once the majority source of donors were relatives; now this has become the exception. However, this technological progress has created a vast range of moral problems. Thirty years ago the

126

moral problem was whether it was right to subject patients to experimental last-resort procedures. Now the moral debate focuses on the inadequate supply of organs and their equitable distribution. For, as the success rate continues, it is inevitable that waiting lists for organs will increase.

A system of distribution which evolved alongside a technology in its infancy is currently under stress in the face of the hopes and aspirations of thousands whose need is obvious and urgent. By the end of 1986 the total number of patients in Europe on dialysis was over 71,000 and it is estimated that the total number of new patients requiring kidneys will rise from the current figure of 17,610 to 25,831 per year (Report of the Conference of European Health Ministers, 1987). Caplan (1983) has drawn attention to the gap between supply and demand in the USA. He pointed out how demand for organs had stretched the voluntary system to the limit, leading to a situation where 'medical hucksters now offer to "solve" the problem by importing organs from paid donors overseas' (ibid:24). He spoke of New York City, with 450 patients waiting for six months or more for corneal transplants to restore their sight. The national figure for the USA was 4,000 blind people waiting for corneas. In New York City there was a waiting list of 600 for kidneys, some of whom had been waiting for over six years. Nationwide, the figure was between 6,000 and 10,000. In the UK the average waiting time for kidney transplants is two years, and there are still approximately 3,800 patients on kidney dialysis awaiting transplants. This figure is increasing by 100 each year. If those awaiting heart, lung and liver transplants are included, there is a total urgent waiting list of well over 4,500, which is a situation where demand far exceeds supply. There have been fluctuations in the supply of organs. Between 1973 and 1985 the gap between supply and demand worsened, although it now appears to have reached a steady state. But this is far from satisfactory. For example, according to the Director of the Nuffield Transplant Unit in Edinburgh, whilst in 1987 1,556 kidneys were transplanted in the UK, by December of that year 3,485 patients were still waiting for a new kidney (Chisholm, 1988:1479).

The situation regarding heart transplants is also far from satisfactory. Mr John Dark, Director of the Cardio-Pulmonary Unit at the Freeman Hospital, Newcastle, estimated that 'about 900 people under 55 on transplant waiting lists are dying every year because of an acute shortage of human donors', and that he saw nothing in the much longer history of kidney transplants to suggest the supply of human heart donors would ever be adequate (the *Guardian*, 6 December 1988). On a national basis the UK Transplant Centre estimate that 'one in five of those who need a heart transplant die on the waiting list because of a shortage of donors' (the *Guardian*, 6 December 1988). Approximately 35 per cent of American candidates for a heart transplant die before an organ donor becomes available (New York Task Force, 1988:35).

The recognized shortage of organs has led to several desperate measures, some of which raise matters of serious ethical concern. An account appeared in *The Hastings Center Report* (Anon., 1989:3–4) of a Michigan pathologist who had written to condemned prisoners across America asking them to donate their organs for transplantation upon execution, and in the meanwhile to sign petitions to convince lawmakers to legalize such donations. One practical and ethical problem with this proposal is that many executions are carried out by means of a lethal injection which causes cardio-pulmonary cessation, thus rendering organs unusable. Organs would have to be removed by means of an anaesthetic prior to death, thus making transplant surgeons effectively executioners. Other objections came from the attorneys representing convicted prisoners, who saw it as a potential creation of another vested interest in capital punishment, perhaps encouraging judges and juries to impose death sentences more readily.

In some cases dramatic appeals for donor organs have been made by prominent politicians and celebrities. These may have some effect on an individual basis, but cannot solve the wider problems of resources. In 1983 President Reagan appealed on the radio for a liver donor for an 11-month-old Texan girl. The appeal was successful but the family could not afford to pay for it. Nevertheless, aware that the White House was concerned, Texas legislators passed a bill authorizing funding for *this* transplant and no other. The problem with high-profile media appeals is their discriminatory and arbitrary nature. Although Reagan was personally involved in several individual appeals he consistently resisted the idea of routine Medicaid funding for transplant operations on the grounds that they would cost too much (Weiss, 1985:22).

The shortage of organs is rapidly becoming an international problem. The Chairman of Turkey's Association of Organ Transplant Patients, Mr Dursan Ozsaglam, estimated that 10,000 patients in Turkey are awaiting kidney transplants and an additional

50,000 are suffering chronic kidney diseases (quoted in *The Times*, 25 January 1989).

ALLOCATING ORGANS

A fair and just allocation of transplant organs requires political and ethical imperatives for the efficient management of organ distribution which transcend national boundaries. There are already signs of the phenomenon known as 'medical tourism' whereby patients appear on several waiting lists in different countries thus ensuring an unfair advantage over others on the waiting list. This problem is one facing politicians and health ministers in the countries affected. There have also been suggestions, at a political level, for a medical equivalent of the 'diplomatic bag', whereby organs transported through customs barriers would not have to be subjected to X-ray searches for terrorist weapons. These are clearly some of the political problems of organ transplantation.

The problem of obtaining an equitable system of allocating organs has not been solved. This is a problem which extends far beyond the scope of transplant ethics, for it involves the essential problem of a fair distribution of medical resources. Most methods of rationing resources have encountered criticism, none perhaps as much as the so-called 'God Committees' in the USA, of which the most widely discussed was the screening process for kidney patients at the Seattle Artificial Kidney Center, whose decisions to allocate scarce resources in the early days of renal dialysis were based, to a certain extent, on a notion of 'social worth', of which in practice the least offensive charge was that it exalted middle class values. Critics have pointed out that it assumed that scout leadership, Red-Cross activities, and religious and social teaching were eternal verities! Public funding helped to resolve the ethical problems of allocating access to the life-saving dialysis programme, but the same problems have re-emerged in the 'tragic choices' now associated with the distribution of hearts and livers.

Policy decisions concerning the allocation of scarce resources, such as transplant organs, rest on two socio-political principles which can be referred to as social utility and egalitarian principles respectively. Decisions to allocate organs on the basis of a social utility principle often invoke a utilitarian framework within which the assessment of a candidate's social worth will be made with reference to his or her capacity to benefit society. Problems arise when one considers the mechanisms required for the evaluation of social worth. How does one weigh up the benefits to society when choosing between an irritating and socially divisive person, like Socrates, and a politician devoted to compromise and stability? So far none of the mechanisms designed to evaluate social worth, in areas other than medicine, has satisfactorily escaped accusations of abuse. It follows that there are no compelling reasons for the introduction of such unsatisfactory practices into already controversial areas in medicine. It might be replied that failure, so far, to construct mechanisms for evaluating social worth is an insufficient reason to conclude that they cannot be created. This objection may be correct. But there are good reasons to suspect that the cost of perfecting such mechanisms could well overtake the cost of providing that very increase in provision of the therapy which would eliminate the need for rationing.

In practice all attempts to single out certain patients as worthy or unworthy of therapy on moral, social, or any other extra-medical grounds, risk accusations of bias, subjectivity and downright corruption. For this reason arguments that liver transplants should be withheld on other than therapeutic grounds from those with alcohol abuse should be resisted lest they introduce a yardstick of moral worthiness.

It is also difficult to apply a principle for withholding therapy which is grounded in the belief that the patient has contributed to his or her condition. This principle could easily apply to the majority of diseased states. And if the principle were endorsed in the case of organ transplants then why should it not be extended to other forms of therapy? Guidelines for withholding therapy on extra-medical grounds are particularly prone to subjectivity, bias and prejudice, and should be avoided altogether, although in certain cases, psycho-social criteria may have to be used when considering transplantation, since a level of mental competence may be required to enable co-operation with the post-operative drug regimen. But stringent efforts must be made to ensure that such criteria are not linked to notions of social worth.

The case for a fundamental egalitarian approach was made soon after the transplant programme began, and it is worth repeating: 'When mortals are called on to make ultimate choices for life and death among their innocent fellows, the only tolerable criterion may be equality of worth as a human being' (Freund, 1971:637). Nevertheless, egalitarian principles generate problems in actual practice. It is difficult to maintain principles of equality when there is not enough to go around. The allocation of organs by means of a lottery is one suggestion in keeping with egalitarian principles, but the objection that such practices are undignified is hard to overcome. The first come first served principle reflects an egalitarian approach, but critics point out that waiting lists are prone to abuse by queue-jumpers. If, however, egalitarian principles are preferable, then queue-jumpers may be the necessary price for equality and fairness in principle, if not always in practice.

Desperate life-and-death situations, nevertheless, will involve desperate strategies, and competition for scarce medical resources is no exception. The high cost of liver transplants is a good example. Weiss (1985:21) recounts a case of a young Massachusetts woman who needed a new liver but both her insurance company and Medicaid refused to pay the $180,000 bill. In this case her father knew someone in the White House who worked as an aide to Ronald Reagan. The presidential aide was contacted and he phoned the Governor of Massachusetts, telling him that unless he convinced Medicaid to reverse their decision he would take out a full page advertisement in a leading newspaper saying 'The Governor of Massachusetts is Responsible for My Daughter's Death'. Medicaid agreed to pay. Unfortunately a suitable donor was not found and the young woman died.

Transplantation of hearts, lungs and livers is expensive because it is labour-intensive. There are frequent objections that a transplantation programme can divert funds from other areas where greater benefit could be obtained for the same cost. Critics frequently draw attention to the high cost of organ transplantation when millions do not have access to basic health care. They complain, with some justification, that media coverage of highly dramatic transplants such as heart–lungs or liver transplants gives high-profile medical teams an unfair advantage over routine therapists in the competition for resources. Frequently, these objections are framed in a utilitarian cast, with appeals to policies aimed at the promotion of the greatest benefit for the greatest number. On a superficial level this could be interpreted in terms of a principle of equality – the maximization of the interests of a majority of equals.

In practice, however, utilitarian systems of distribution raise serious problems concerning fairness and equity. In a commentary on a decision by a US authority to transfer funds from a child's liver transplant operation to another area of need, Franklin (1988:36) drew attention to this case as an example of utilitarianism's 'inherent potential for discrimination, the possibility that what is perceived as "good" for the majority may be bad for the minority'. As a matter of principle society would not allow children to be injected with live AIDS virus if one child in a hundred developed the disease, even if the majority developed immunity. For this reason, maintained Franklin:

> when we consider the plight of the child who dies without an organ transplant because funding has been rerouted to a 'greater good' we are in fact witnessing the discriminatory aspect of utilitarianism. . . . In the case of organ transplants, government policy would perpetuate an already de facto discriminatory system.
>
> (ibid:35)

It is unfortunate, but true, that most societies practise various forms of discrimination. Utilitarian appeals to the greater good simply reinforce this. 'It is well documented,' says Franklin, 'that the indigent, certain racial groups, and those with less access to the media are less likely to receive organ transplants. The negative consequences of such rationing are unambiguous – these people will die' (ibid:35).

In the UK fears are often expressed that patients in the private sector may be given priority over NHS patients and spend a shorter time on waiting lists. These fears are regularly rebutted by officials but they are based on long-standing beliefs in class inequality and privilege. Moreover, it has been pointed out that whilst there is a two-year waiting list for kidney transplants 'doctors appear to have a large amount of discretion over the urgency of particular cases' in particular over judgements concerning depression incurred by prolonged dialysis or judgements concerning tissue matching (the *Guardian*, 2 February 1989). Mr Ross Taylor, a consultant transplant surgeon at the Royal Victoria Hospital, Newcastle, was reported to have said (the *Guardian*, 7 February 1989) that there was nothing to stop a doctor from taking a kidney intended for one of the 3,700 people on the waiting list for transplants to allow one of his private patients to jump the queue. There are also about 50 kidneys each year which become available from the USA for the UK private sector. These are due to alleged inefficiencies in the USA system of distribution and a reluctance by USA physicians to use kidneys over 24 hours old. Stories frequently appear in USA newspapers that some transplant centres have passed over Americans waiting for a donated liver, heart or kidney, to transplant foreign nationals willing to make large donations to the medical centre (New York Task Force, 1988:116). Whether or not each charge of queue-jumping by wealthy private patients can be substantiated there is a widespread consensus among the public and medical personnel that such a practice is morally reprehensible.

If equality, rather than selectivity and privilege, is a guiding principle then the weight of urgent moral concern should be concentrated on tolerable methods to increase the availability of transplant organs and resources to facilitate transplantation procedures.

Throughout Europe and the USA the principles governing organ collection are based on informed consent and voluntarism. These principles are closely related to beliefs in the autonomy of rational adults, the value of altruism as a social good and respect for the person. When evaluating various options for meeting a scarcity of transplant organs the above-mentioned principles and beliefs will function as the framework within which such discourse can take place.

ORGAN PROCUREMENT

Options for obtaining transplant organs can be considered under five categories:

(1) buying and selling,
(2) trading,
(3) taking,
(4) giving, and
(5) requesting.

Buying and selling

There are legal prohibitions governing the sale of organs from living donors throughout Europe, the USA, and most of the world, although there have been widely discussed cases of live organ sales in India, and several arguments in favour of a market

133

approach to the supply of required organs have appeared in recent Anglo-American philosophy journals.

On 25 December 1983 the following advertisement appeared in the Burlington County issue of the *New Jersey Times*:

KIDNEY FOR SALE
From 32 yr. old Caucasian
female in excellent health
Write to P.O. Box ...
NJ 085

This was not an isolated case. A man in Georgia offered to sell a kidney for $25,000 to buy a fast food restaurant. But then came competition. A woman in the state offered one of her kidneys at a knockdown price of $5,000. Meanwhile, the rate in California was higher – some would-be kidney vendors were asking up to $160,000 (Weiss, 1985:17). A more ambitious scheme was proposed in 1983 by an American, Dr H. Barry Jacobs, who attempted to found an International Kidney Exchange, which would buy organs from around the world and sell them at a higher price to those who wanted them. Though not illegal at the time the plan was strongly denounced by the US National Kidney Foundation as 'immoral and unethical'. It did not take much imagination to see how such a plan would benefit the wealthy countries at the expense of the poor. When the US Congress denounced the plan, Albert Gove, Senator from Tennessee, said: 'People should not be regarded as things to be bought and sold like parts of an automobile' (ibid:20).

One of the strongest objections to the sale of organs is a version of the slippery slope argument expressed in the Report of the Conference of European Health Ministers in November 1987, which stated:

If there is nothing unethical about the removal of an organ from a living person, is there not a danger that pressure might one day be brought to bear on a possible donor 'for good of the nation' or even 'for the good of mankind'? could forget the criminal excesses to which this disre- for the human person can lead? To ensure that the n of an organ is not tainted in any way, the physician able to satisfy himself that it is totally spontaneous etely without payment. Yet how can one be sure

134

that no pressure – there are many different kinds – has been brought to bear on the donor? How can one tell that the apparently voluntary donor has not derived any profit from what appears to be a disinterested gift? What doctor would dare to vouch for what may happen behind the scenes? The sale of human organs is no longer a myth and the wealthiest can buy life at the expense of the most underprivileged. That is where we have been led by an act of which ethics approves, and we are only at the beginning of a venture frought with dangers. Organ donation is undoubtedly a profoundly humane gesture, but its legislation and use without major restrictions involve one of the greatest risks man has ever run: that of giving a value to his body, a price to his life. Very many countries, be they poor or very rich, are also confronted with the increasing development of an organ market, whatever the ostensible ethics and whatever the legislation.

(Report of the Conference of European Health Ministers, 1987:15)

In the above passage is a very serious warning of a slippery slope which may start with unregulated organ removal and end with a vicious traffic whereby the poor and the uneducated would be exploited in the interest of the wealthy.

Arguments in favour of organ sales usually reflect a belief in the alleged inherent efficiency of market transactions. There have been various proposals for a market in cadaver organs, whereby sales could be conducted either by relatives or by means of a prior arrangement with the deceased. However, the sale of cadaveric organs is prohibited in European and most other countries by laws which prohibit the ownership of dead bodies for commercial profit. Arguments in favour of a market solution to the problems of organ allocation should be treated with caution. There is little evidence to support the view that market forces are capable of providing an equitable distribution of commodities and payment for labour, an area where there has been considerable experience over many years. On the so far unsuccessful past record of market forces one should be wary of proposals to extend them as a solution to problems in the relatively new area of organ allocation. One objection to proposals for a market approach to organ procurement is that, if legalized, the sale of organs would merely reflect the low moral standing of a social system that reduced people to that kind of action. Critics have pointed out that it is inherently inequitable and undermines society's commitment to fundamental values of justice and fairness. It would take little imagination to predict how organ sales would favour the wealthy at the expense of the poor, among whom many could be forced into a sub-class of involuntary donors. Even the suggestion that tax reductions for organ donors would encourage altruism has a hollow ring once it is recognized that it makes the organs of the rich more valuable than those of the poor.

Another variation on the theme of organ selling is the proposal to encourage organ donation by giving in exchange credits or units to offset costs which may be incurred when a family member requires organs. The objection here is that it contravenes the principle of equality of access to life-sustaining therapy. Other variations include proposals to reimburse organ donors rather than pay them outright for their organs. There is little to be said for this argument. The line between reimbursement and payment is extremely hard to maintain, and for the desperately poor reimbursement could well be seized upon as eagerly as payment.

It has been argued that precedents for a market in live organs have been set by the sale, in the USA and several other countries, of blood and sperm. But these are replaceable and, under appropriate conditions, involve little or no risk to the seller. The sale of vital non-regenerating organs would constitute various forms of assault on the seller. One might pay someone to sit an examination in one's place, which is both immoral and illegal, but involves no physical harm. But there are serious moral objections against paying someone to put themselves in mortal danger for us. This is even worse if it involves trading on that person's poverty.

Nevertheless, pressure for organs will lead to corruption until morally acceptable alternative solutions are found. Before advances in dental mechanics facilitated adequate false dentures rich patients in the eighteenth century paid for teeth wrenched out of the mouths of the poor for unsuccessful transplants. The shortage of cadavers for medical dissection in the nineteenth century encouraged Burke and Hare to follow the profit motive from grave robbing to murder. This gruesome episode of entrepreneurship did not end in the nineteenth century. Throughout the world are reports of a hidden market in organs where wealthy clients benefit at the expense of the poor. Jonsen (1988:246) cites instances in the USA of 'individuals, particularly wealthy foreigners, who have moved to the top of waiting lists for transplants and pay almost four times the amount charged to citizens'. In Hong Kong today there are reports of sales of kidneys extracted from executed criminals in Canton (the *Guardian*, 7 February 1989). There have also been several reports of payments of around £3,000 to kidney donors from the Indian sub-continent who have passed themselves off as relatives of recipients in the UK. When allegations were made by two Turkish peasants that they had been paid £2,000 each, plus expenses, to travel from Turkey to be live kidney donors in a private hospital in London, there was an outcry in the British media and an immediate investigation (*The Times*, 23 January 1989; the *Guardian* 23 and 24 January 1989). This led to a speed-up of plans by the Royal College of Surgeons for a computer register of all organs donated and received in the UK (the *Guardian*, 28 January 1989) and a decision by the British Government to pass legislation to outlaw organ sales.

Although it was not illegal in the UK until 1989 to carry out an operation on a donor who has been paid for an organ, health ministers acting on behalf of the British Government had made it clear in 1985 that they were opposed to such a practice and would withhold the licence from any private hospital which carried out such an operation. The sale of organs is opposed by the General Medical Council, which published a statement in November 1985, stressing that it was unethical for any doctor to be involved in any way in the trafficking of human organs. The Council of the Transplantation Society has opposed the sale of kidneys by live donors, a view shared by the British Transplantation Society. Moreover, the Government of the UK is party to a Council of Europe resolution condemning the commercialization of human organs. A junior health minister described the practice as 'improper, undesirable, and unacceptable' (the *Guardian*, 24 January 1989). The need for urgent but well thought out legislation on this issue has long been overdue.

Nevertheless, two arguments in favour of organ sales have been advanced, and will be considered here. First, it has been argued that the sale of organs would increase the supply. This may be the case, but an increase in supply is not an adequate moral reason for adopting a proposal on organ provision. Supplies could also be increased by drafting individuals at random, or by compulsorily dissecting mental patients and, no doubt, many other reprehensible means could be found.

The second argument takes the form of an appeal to the individual's liberty over his or her body. This argument was recently employed by a West German businessman whose attempt to launch a European market for kidney sales from a British base was reported on Central TV (ITV News, 29 January 1989). He described the potential clients as 'businessmen who have a certain standard of living which they wish to keep or improve and who are willing to sell a kidney to achieve it' (the *Guardian*, 30 January 1989). On these terms the sale of human organs is no different to the sale of any other commodity that a vendor exercises a right to dispose of. But this again is an appeal without substance. In some of the freest societies in the world there are limits on the liberty one can exercise over one's body. These might include prostitution, limits on abortion, limits on boxers who fail to meet health standards, health and safety regulations at work and participation in dangerous experiments.

The arguments against selling organs are overwhelming. It reflects a commodification of bodies, a dilution of altruism, and it fails to meet both logical and economic objections. For example, voluntary consent to sale would be self-refuting as the organs would come from those who (a) were economically coerced, (b) had a hopelessly misguided perception regarding the transaction, or (c) were reasonably wealthy but obsessively concerned with accumulating money at any price. None of these categories should be considered as an acceptable basis for the distribution of transplant organs.

Trading, exchange and distribution

Trading or exchanging organs exists on a rather *ad hoc* basis either among hospitals within a country or across national frontiers. Apart from many loose and informal structures several organ-exchange organizations exist. Centralized cadaveric transplantation was a possibility due to the national health systems of several European countries. In Europe there is Eurotransplant, an international organ exchange programme that utilizes tissue-typing methods. There is also France transplant, Hispano transplant, LUSO transplant, North Italy transplant, Scandia transplant, Swiss transplant and UK transplant. Eurotransplant was set up in 1967 to distribute organs in Holland, Belgium, Austria and part of West Germany. Scandia transplant was set up in 1969 to share organs in Norway, Sweden, and Denmark. The UK and Switzerland created national organ sharing systems in the 1970s. These exchange organizations function primarily as vehicles for improving the exchange of donor organs and ensuring the most suitable recipients. Apart from organizational procedures dealing with organ procurement through to transplant operations they play a liaison role between laboratories, donor, and transplant centres. They keep registers of potential donors and recipients, attempt to formulate methods for improving the donor–recipient match to overcome rejection problems, and generally seek to create a donor pool of significant size to facilitate compatible donor–recipient matching. To this end, every exchange organization maintains a computerized waiting list. Since the early 1970s the European exchange organizations have circulated a 'list of urgent cases' with regard to the urgent provision of kidney grafts.

Facilities for national integrated methods of distribution have been rather slow to develop. But recent developments are more optimistic. In the UK local registers of potential donors have been organized in major cities, such as Cardiff, Manchester, Glasgow, and Birmingham. In each of these cities a computer-based register has been initiated, to which local ICUs have access. The long-term intention is that they will become the forerunners of a national network. In the USA, the National Organ Transplant Act of 1984, subsequently amended in 1986 and 1988, formed the basis of a national USA distributors' policy for transplant organs, together with the setting up of an Organ Procurement and Transplantation Network with the objective of compiling a single national list of patients awaiting transplants, assessed in terms of medical urgency.

In 1988 a report from the New York State Task Force on Life and the Law urged state action to reform existing USA organ procurement and distribution agencies, recommending the creation of an executive Transplant Council, the adoption of uniform criteria for donor suitability, regulation of procurement agencies, and the development of a universal patient list for extra-renal organs (New York Task Force, 1988). There are no plans at present for a world-wide list, or even a single European list.

Until recently most international arrangements for organ exchange have been informal, often based on personal contacts among the surgeons involved. One encouraging aspect of inter-national trade took place in June 1979. Following the death of a 14-year-old American girl in Norfolk, Virginia, both her kidneys were removed for possible transplantation. But because the anti-gens of her kidneys were of an unusual combination, no American recipient was found on the waiting list, so the search was extended to Italy, Kuwait and Russia. Eventually a patient was located in Moscow and the kidney was flown out there and was successfully transplanted. Three weeks later a pair of kidneys arrived from Russia under similar circumstances (Varga, 1984:215).

Routine taking and presumed consent

Laws which facilitate routine taking, or presumed consent, empower physicians or coroners to remove organs or tissues from a deceased patient without the prior expressed consent of the patient. In several countries the presumption of consent is over-come if the family object to the donation. In the USA many states have enacted laws authorizing the removal of corneas and pituitary glands on a presumed consent basis, but do not extend this to the removal of solid organs, such as hearts, lungs, kidneys and livers. Public opinion surveys in the USA indicate widespread opposition to routine taking (New York Task Force, 1988:25). On the other hand in Austria, Czechoslovakia, Denmark, France, Israel, Poland, and Switzerland, solid organs can be procured on a presumed consent basis. The wide range of statutes and practices concerning presumed consent are indicative of a lack of consensus regarding donation, and a need for greater assimilation of the ethical signifi-cance of organ transplantation.

Taking, or routine salvaging of organs, would save many lives and alleviate any shortage of organs reducing costs and time spent in the search for voluntary donors. Those in favour of routine taking argue that it would avoid making awkward and very often painful requests to distressed relatives, and would eliminate the effort of carrying donor cards and save valuable time which is currently spent in looking for them. In the UK there are annually about 4,000 patients in ICUs who are diagnosed as brain dead. Owing to unsuitability and lack of consent only between a fifth and a half of kidneys from patients diagnosed as brain dead were used in Britain in 1987 (Chisholm, 1988:1479).

The major ethical problem concerning routine salvaging is not,

140

strictly speaking, over the mutilation of the corpse, as most religious and secular moral systems acknowledge that organs can be removed under appropriate conditions. The question is whether organs should be removed without prior consent. There are, however, precedents. In most Western countries post-mortems are conducted without consent, often for seemingly trivial reasons, and this practice does not appear to offend relatives and society in general. If organs can be removed for post-mortem enquiries then why not for the purpose of transplantation? Objections usually appeal to the loss of autonomy (Lamb, 1988) and the opportunity to exercise generosity (Ramsey, 1970). If organ donation is one of the supreme gifts that one individual can bestow on another, it is argued, society cannot afford to lose such altruistic practices, the benefits of which spread further than the demand for more transplantable organs.

Most of the arguments in favour of routine taking of solid organs are utilitarian and are based on an appeal to a favourable balance of lives saved. This policy could be implemented, so it is argued, with provisions for opting out arrangements for those with religious or moral objections. Routine taking, on these terms, could be seen to incorporate an element of consent in that an individual who has not expressed a wish to the contrary may be presumed to have consented to donation. This is sometimes referred to as a 'contracting out' or 'opting out' arrangement. At present 13 of the 21 member states of the Council of Europe have legislation in favour of presumed consent. The underlying assumptions guiding proposals for presumed consent are based on observations that during the donor's lifetime he or she never expressed objections to organ removal and that there were no indications of religious or philosophical or moral convictions against the use of his or her organs for transplantation. In 1978 France adopted a system of contracting out, whereby it became legal to transplant organs from the recently dead unless he/she had signed a special register forbidding the removal of organs after death. Finland, Greece, Italy, Norway, Spain and Sweden have laws based on presumed consent, but physicians consult with relatives. In Austria, Czechoslovakia, Denmark, France, Israel, Poland and Switzerland, physicians may proceed without asking the next of kin, unless a prior objection has been raised by the family of the deceased. Belgium has recently introduced a system whereby all those wishing to opt out may do so at the offices of their local authority. Those who do not register are presumed to have consented.

The arguments in favour of presumed consent sometimes rest on a form of tacit social contract theory. It is argued that some countries have now reached a stage of development that allows their populations to have at their disposal sufficient information on the beneficial effects of organ transplantation. Under such circumstances it can be presumed that individuals would have made their objections known during their lifetime.

One of the objections to presumed consent is that the application of presumption is gratuitous when there is no sure way of checking that presumption. It is also argued that the presumption in favour of donation will lead to a situation where the poor, the uneducated, and the legally disenfranchized might bear a disadvantageous burden, and only the more advantaged groups would exercise autonomy.

The objections are usually based on a version of the slippery slope argument; namely the prediction that it would lead to a cheapening of respect for human life, where patients near to death are viewed as potential resource banks. There are also implications whereby the state, or some agency empowered by the state, would be granted extensive powers over human remains.

In 1979 British transplant surgeon, Robert Sells, argued against any change in the direction of an opting out policy on the grounds that 'the present law is ... sufficiently unrestrictive to allow legally sanctioned removal of organs from people who die in hospital; and more important, the supply of organs for transplantation would not be significantly increased by changing the law to an opting out principle' (Sells, 1979:165). He reported that as high as 94 per cent acceptance by relatives was achieved if they were approached by the transplant team, although when 'donors' doctors interview the relatives the refusal rate may be higher' (ibid:168). On these terms it would be unnecessary to introduce new laws and any shift in principle away from voluntary donation. Sells also emphasized how a high acceptance rate was bound up with treating relatives with respect, acknowledging their willingness to see the benefits of donation. Much of this good will could be lost if routine salvaging were adopted. He also stressed the importance of maintaining contact with medical personnel responsible for the donor; that the transplant team should notify doctors and nurses concerned with the donor of the results of the transplant. 'This simple act of good manners,' wrote Sells, 'will probably result in more donors being referred' (ibid:168). Given the high acceptance rates and maintenance of good will, any endorsement of a contracting out system would require evidence that relatives were not being approached or that a significant number were objecting. The first reason could be dealt with by ensuring better means of contact with relatives, whereas the latter is clearly not a good reason for changing as it would be perceived as a tyrannical step.

The problem of requesting organs from distressed relatives should not be underestimated. A great deal of understanding, tact and empathy is required at a time when transplant surgeons have urgent duties to the potential recipient. The case in favour of contracting out is often advanced as a partial solution to this problem. The British MP, Tam Dalyell, has tried (so far unsuccessfully) several times to introduce a bill (The Human Organs Bill) in Parliament with contracting out provisions. His proposal entailed a computerized list of those who object to organ removal. A phone call to the computer would then determine whether the person had contracted out and risky delays would be eliminated. Apart from the benefits of more organs Dalyell sought to alleviate the unease of doctors and surgeons who, at a time of maximum grief, have to ask relatives 'Can we have the organs of your loved one?'. 'How many of us', asked Dalyell, 'would have the heart to put to a shattered mother or father or a young wife such a question within minutes of their hearing, for example, of a motor smash?' Yet in these situations time is limited and Dalyell's proposal would save time. Thus 'if the question is delayed, the organ deteriorates and becomes less useful to someone in need' (Dalyell, 1974).

Any steps that avoid additional grief in such distressing circumstances are surely to be welcomed. Dalyell's proposal would certainly alleviate anxiety amongst medical personnel, and there is much to be said for that. But would it alleviate the distress of the relatives concerned? On Dalyell's scenario relatives, on hearing of the emergency, rush to the hospital to be almost simultaneously told of the death, or impending death, of their loved one and asked to authorize the removal of organs. But an equally distressing scenario could be described under a contracting out system. Within minutes of hearing about the accident relatives rush to the hospital to be told: 'We've checked through the computer, she hadn't contracted out, so we have begun to remove her heart, lungs, kidneys, eyes, and. . . .' If this scenario is plausible it would seem that intrusion into grief arguments cancel each other out, and that the case for or against presumed consent must be settled on other grounds.

Given that respect for the individual is one of the cornerstones of medical ethics, to weaken an individual's power of direction – even the power to direct some events after one's death – is seen as an attack on this cornerstone. As Veatch argues:

> If the body is essential to the individual's identity in a society which values personal integrity and freedom, it must be the individual's first of all to control, not only over a life-time, but within reasonable limits after that life has gone as well. If the body is to be made available to others for personal and societal research, it must be a gift.
>
> (Veatch, 1976:268–9)

Foremost critics of both routine salvaging and presumed consent as well as Veatch include the Protestant theologian, Paul Ramsey (1970), and Leon Kass (1985), who argue that it is coercive and could result in an abuse of the civil rights of religious minorities who oppose the 'mutilation' of dead bodies. In the USA and the UK at present, public policy is tipped towards voluntarism, recognizing the legal status of donor cards, and rights of the next of kin to make decisions on behalf of deceased relatives. Such voluntarism, it is argued, encourages social virtues of the kind outlined in Richard Titmus's *The Gift Relationship* (1971). In this context the practice of blood donation in the UK is frequently cited as an example of public generosity. So far all of the proposed bills for establishing presumed consent with contracting out arrangements have been unsuccessful in the UK. Nevertheless, pressure for change in this direction remains and failure to support such measures in the light of an increasing need for organ transplants has been described as a 'less than charitable attempt on the part of the Government and the rest of us to slough this particular problem on to doctors' (Kennedy, 1988:255).

Giving

Organs can be donated either by prior direction of the deceased or by the family responsible for disposal of the person's remains.

144

In the USA the Uniform Anatomical Gift Act (UAGA), which has been widely adopted, authorizes an individual to donate his body, organs, or tissue, for the purpose of transplantation or other scientific use, by means of a simple witnessed document. Alternatively the Act empowers the next of kin (in order of priority, beginning with the spouse) to grant authorization. Several millions of American citizens carry UAGA cards. In the UK the system is primarily voluntary and donor cards can be easily obtained, but the legal basis of organ donation has been accused of ambiguity (Kennedy, 1988:242–3). The earliest legal guidelines in the UK can be found in the 1952 Corneal Grafting Act which was the first statute dealing directly with the transplantation of tissue. This was repealed in 1961 when the Human Tissue Act made provisions generally for cadaveric transplants without reference to specific tissue or organs. The alleged ambiguity in the guidelines it provided concerning donation can be seen in the following description. The Act endorses the deceased's express view to donate, which means that the element of consent is considered as express consent, as opposed to the presumed consent (which was considered under the category of taking). But in the absence of a view expressed by the deceased, it would seem that a form of presumed consent is operative subject to a veto by spouse or relatives.

In several countries express consent can be conditioned by third parties, such as relatives, who may override the deceased's wishes in certain circumstances. But one of the central problems here turns on the family's alleged right to veto the previously recorded wishes of the deceased. In Ireland, the Netherlands and Spain the wishes of the family are legally recognized to have priority over both the expressed and the presumed wishes of the deceased. However, it appears, as a matter of consistency at least, that if we uphold the right not to donate, as a right which cannot be vetoed, then the right to donate without veto should also exist. In so far as the wishes of the family ought to be taken into consideration it would appear that the exercise of a family veto should be given less weight in cases of express consent. For in the latter case it is the legal right of the deceased to will donation that must be weighed against whatever reason the family may have for refusing donation. In the case of presumed consent, a case could be made for giving greater weight to the family's objections.

There is, however, a serious question mark over the relatives' decision to donate the organs of the deceased. Do they, in reality, freely consent? Consider the situation in which relatives are approached. Usually the potential donor has died suddenly and unexpectedly. The most suitable donors are young people who die from massive head injuries. The relatives are in a state of shock and grief. This is not the most perfect situation for making calm and rational decisions. Moreover, the capacity of the bereaved to comprehend information is always questionable. Even when they later claim that they made the correct decision at the time one can still see this as a rationalization. Then there is the role of the physician. How close to deception does he or she travel when deciding whether to paint an optimistic picture of the potential success and benefits derived from removal, or whether to downplay the possibility of rejection? In these circumstances it is extremely difficult to maintain a strict distinction between encouragement to donate and pressure or coercion. Yet on this distinction rests the case against routine salvaging or presumed consent.

It is in this context that the reluctance of medical personnel to approach relatives should be considered. There is genuine resistance to appearing 'ghoulish', even when the motives are clearly commendable. But as we have seen, the adoption of a contracting out system will not resolve this problem. One suggestion might alleviate distress in this situation: relatives should not be approached with a request for organs until they have been informed that the patient has been pronounced dead. There must be no element of fudge here. A ventilated brainstem dead patient is a cadaver, and relatives should not be confused by references to irreversible coma and states which are as 'good as dead' or explanations to the effect that 'it's only the machines that are keeping her alive'. The case for delaying requests for organs has been argued convincingly by Annas (1988) who stresses the separation of criteria for brain death and organ donation:

> It is essential that no request for organs be made until *after* the patient is pronounced dead; if the request is refused, the body should be immediately released to the family. Making requests prior to the announcement of death leads not only to real conflicts of interest (between treating the patient as a person and as an organ source) but also to ... suffering and confusion. ... It could also reinforce the two primary

reasons the public gives for not signing donor cards: fear that doctors 'might do something to me before I'm really dead' and fear that 'doctors might hasten my death'.

(Annas, 1988:29)

Opinion polls repeatedly indicate public support for organ donation, despite the fact that relatively few members of the public carry donor cards. A Gallup poll in the *Guardian*, 30 December 1988, revealed 85 per cent opinion in favour of transplants. The same year the British Kidney Patients Association conducted an opinion poll which indicated 70 per cent of respondents willing to donate, but only 29 per cent possessed donor cards. Given this extent of public support a case for routine taking with presumed consent could be advanced. It could also be argued that pressure to donate should not be applied to a minority of families at the time of bereavement, and that at least routine taking (with contracting out arrangements) would spread this pressure more evenly.

It may be impossible to reach a clear-cut decision in favour of either policies based on taking organs (with presumed consent) or policies based on giving (express consent). It would seem that two levels of argument are employed and need to be distinguished. At one level are the practical arguments based on the need for organs and the beneficial consequences of increasing the harvest. The decision here between taking and giving would simply turn on which side presented the most convincing argument for the strategy which could maximize supply. If the sole criterion is a policy that will maximize the number of organs under the most efficient methods then contracting out is the most satisfactory strategy, provided there are safeguards to minimize distress caused to relatives. But on another level are conflicts which may only be resolved by a general shift in the moral climate. For it is impossible to weigh up and assess arguments which counter the interests of the dead and the living. Those who oppose routine salvaging of organs express concern for matters such as the integrity of the corpse (recognizing its symbolic role), the emotional feelings of the relatives, and notions of respect for the being that was. Opponents who dismiss these objections as lingering forms of emotional immaturity have not even begun to address these issues, which go deep into the heart of most of the world's cultures.

Request

A method which could be a compromise between contracting in and contracting out of organ donation is the system of 'routine inquiry' or routine request, which has operated in the USA since 1986. According to this doctrine hospitals are under an obligation to request relatives of dying patients to consider organ donation *after* the death of the patient in question. Quite obviously such a course, if universally adopted, would require methods of disseminating more detailed counselling skills to the physicians and hospital personnel whose task it is to inform relatives about death or impending death. The reluctance of physicians in some quarters to embrace required request is obviously understandable. However, part of this burden is shifted from the doctors by placing responsibility for requiring on the hospitals. So far 38 states in the USA have enacted legislation requiring hospitals to make routine enquiries about potential organ donation, seeking information whether donation would be approved by the next of kin. In the autumn of 1987 required request became federal law. As a condition of participation in the Medicare and Medicaid programme, each US hospital is required to have written protocols to ensure routine informing of such families and informing of a federal certified organ procurement agency when a potential donor is available. A request is not required if the hospital has prior notice of the decedent's or relatives' objection to donation, or there is a reason to believe that organ donation is contrary to the decedent's religious beliefs. It is predicted that these arrangements will greatly enlarge the supply of donor organs and help optimize their distribution. But is it enough? As two US transplant surgeons commented: 'it will be unlikely to meet the overall demands for cardiac donors' (Schroeder and Hunt, 1987:3143).

In the UK required request was considered by the DHSS, but was rejected in favour of a policy involving better information concerning donation and an extension of the donor card system. Nevertheless, it could be argued that required request might be one way of closing the gap between voluntary donors and patients requiring organs. One estimate in the USA suggests that whilst 200,000 persons are declared brain dead each year, organs are only harvested from 2,000, whilst the combined need for hearts, lungs, and kidneys, is estimated at 50,000 or more (Schwartz, 1985). In the UK there are an estimated 4,000 cases where brainstem criteria determine death, which could alleviate some of the pressure of the 3,800 awaiting kidney transplants and the 500 awaiting heart transplants.

CONCLUSION

It would seem that if pressure for organs increases then arguments in favour of either presumed consent, with opting out arrangements, or required request, would be the best alternatives to a wholly voluntary system. If a voluntary system is to be maintained it clearly must attract more voluntary organ donors which in turn partly rests upon achieving greater public confidence in the definitions of and criteria for brainstem death. In this respect the media (at least in the UK) lags behind medical facts and philosophical theory in its periodic scaremongering reports of reversals of brain death and its occasional portrayal of transplant surgeons as organ vultures. These fears may certainly explain the paradoxical discrepancy between opinion polls in favour of organ donation and the relatively small number of those possessing donor cards. In several countries widespread support has not been translated into higher procurement rates. Following adverse reports on brain death criteria in the UK there was a 20 per cent drop in organ donations as recently as the first three months of 1987. Then again, in the early months of 1989, following reports of kidney sales in a private hospital in London, there was a drop in the number of donors of hearts and kidneys. According to one calculation up to 100 people may have died as a result. Professor Ben Bradley, Director of the UK Transplant Service, which co-ordinates transplants nationally, attributed this decline in donor rates to the reports of kidney sales which had 'unjustifiably shaken the public's confidence in transplantation' (the *Guardian*, 29 May 1989).

To counter these periodic bouts of public disenchantment and apathy better methods of publicizing the need for donors are necessary. Efforts have recently been made in this direction. British Telecom, in 1988, distributed four million donor cards with telephone bills in the London area. In the first three months of 1988 three million donor cards were accepted in the UK. And to publicize the need for heart donors special US basketball teams, consisting of heart transplant patients, have played matches with donor cards being distributed to spectators. Other proposals, now

149

in force in the USA, include provisions for individuals to express consent to organ donation on their driving licence, or to register as a donor when they apply for a new licence. In September of 1989 over 400 transplant recipients took part in the World Transplant Games in Singapore. Other proposals include the setting up of 'transplant days' in hospitals, held once a year, when members of the public can meet transplant surgeons and organ recipients. There is also a need for better information about the mechanics of brainstem death in nursing and medical courses.

There is a need, too, for further investigation into reasons why potential sources are not adequately used. Here, an understanding of the symbolic role of the dead body has to be appreciated. Pressure for multi-organ donation may contribute to relatives' resistance to accept large-scale harvesting of organs. Reasons often cited for refusal are that the patient 'has been through enough', which suggests notions of psychic or moral, but certainly symbolic, continuity across the boundary between life and death.

The New York Task Force on Life and The Law summarized the three most cited obstacles to donation as follows: '(i) reluctance to contemplate and provide for one's death; (ii) fear that a willingness to donate might lead to premature termination of medical care; and (iii) religious and moral objections to desecration of the body' (New York Task Force, 1988:22).

In the UK recent cuts in hospital funding have been a considerable obstacle. Mr Ross Taylor, president of the British Transplantation Society, said in the *Guardian* (29 May 1989) that 'in some cases doctors were unable to take up valuable operating time, space and staff to carry out the necessary operations to remove organs because hospital budgets were "extremely tight"'. Practical limits on theatre time place a severe restriction on multiple organ retrieval, which may occupy a theatre for hours. This is a clear disincentive to organ procurement, especially when theatres are needed for emergencies. Moreover, a small hospital, which pays overtime for a medical team to remove organs from a brain dead accident victim, receives no recompense from the Government. This might seem trivial, but as one heart transplant surgeon pointed out, 'At a time when everyone is operating on very tight limits, that can make a difference' (the *Guardian*, 6 December 1988).

Intensive care units are potential sources but many patients who might be donors do not get into the units. Some doctors prefer to care for some dying patients on the wards and do not want them started on positive pressure ventilation. This is legitimate, and therapy should not be directed with extrinsic interests in mind, but patients not on ventilators cannot be suitable donors.

As greater awareness of the benefits of organ transplantation filters through into the public mind, as a clearer perception is achieved concerning the extent to which transplants of non-regenerative organs have become part of routine therapy rather than high-risk experiment, so ethical approval of organ transplants is likely to increase. All of this requires a massive effort in public information concerning the opportunities which organ transplants offer and strong reassurances that these opportunities are not at the expense of the weaker members of society.

It should also be stressed that none of the systems of organ procurement is, at present, satisfactory. The sale and purchase of organs is an affront to human altruism and would, from the start, involve exploitation and degradation. Routine salvaging, with presumed consent, might risk overriding an individual's deeply felt objection to post-mortem donation, whilst the operation of a veto by relatives may frustrate a genuine desire to become a donor. In fact none of the systems in practice today can guarantee that an individual's wishes will be respected. The wishes of the donor card holder may be frustrated because no one looked for the card, or the family concealed the fact that one was held. A system of presumed consent might go into operation before it is known that the individual did not wish to donate.

The way forward seems clear. National central registers should be set up consisting of names of donors who have given express consent and those who have indicated a desire not to donate. Every hospital should then have instant access to this register. To avoid incorrect recordings on the register and to allow opportunity to revoke a decision, individuals should be regularly contacted, by letter, to reaffirm (or reconsider) their status. This massive involvement of the public should be developed alongside a well thought out information policy on the benefits of organ transplants, and procurement policies which are compatible with notions of respect for the human body.

BIBLIOGRAPHY

Ad Hoc Committee of the Harvard Medical School (1968) 'A definition of irreversible coma', *Journal of the American Medical Association* 205, 6:85–8.

Anderson, Ian (1989) 'Surgeons transplant liver from living donor', *New Scientist* 12 August:26.

Annas, George, J. (1987) 'From Canada with love: anencephalic newborns as organ donors', *Hastings Center Report* December:36–8.

____(1988) 'Brain death and organ donation: you *can* have one without the other', *Hastings Center Report* June/July:28–30.

Anon. (a) (1989) 'Retinal transplants could be an answer to blindness', *New Scientist* 5 August:25.

____(b) (1989) 'An eye for an eye', *Hastings Center Report* March/-April:3–4.

Arnold, John D., Zimmerman, Thomas F., and Martin, Daniel C. (1968) 'Public attitudes and the diagnosis of death', *Journal of the American Medical Association* 206, 9:1949–54.

Beresford, H.R. (1978) 'Cognitive death: differential problems and legal overtones', *Annals of the New York Academy of Sciences* 315:339–48.

Black, Peter McL. (1978) 'Brain death', *New England Journal of Medicine* 299:338–44 and 211:393–401.

____(1985) 'Predicting the outcome from hypoxic–ischemic coma; medical and ethical implications', *Journal of the American Medical Association* 254, 9:1215–16.

BMA Working Party (1988) 'Conclusions of the BMA Working Party set up to review the association's guidance on euthanasia', *BMJ* 14 May 296:1376–7.

Botkin, Jeffrey, R. (1988) 'Anencephalic infants as organ donors', *Pediatrics*, 82, 2:250–6.

Bradley, B.A. (1988) Letter, *BMJ* 14 May 296:1377.

Browne, A. (1983) 'Whole brain death reconsidered', *Journal of Medical Ethics* 9:28–31.

Calne, Sir Roy (ed.) (1987) *Liver Transplantation*, Orlando: Grune & Stratton.

Caplan, Arthur L. (1983) 'Organ transplantation: the cost of success', *Hastings Center Report* Dec.:23–32.

——(1987) 'Should fetuses or infants be used as organ donors?' *Bioethics* 1:119–40.

Capron, Alexander Morgan (1987) 'Anencephalic donors: separate the dead from the dying', *Hastings Center Report* Feb.:5–8.

——(1988) 'The report of the President's Commission on the uniform declaration of death act', in Richard M. Zaner (ed.) *Death: Beyond Whole-Brain Criteria*, Dordrecht: Kluwer, 147–69.

Carse, James P. (1978) 'The social effects of changing attitudes about death', *Annals of the New York Academy of Science* 315:322–38.

Chisholm, Geoffrey B. (1988) 'Time to end softly softly approach on harvesting organs for transplantation', *BMJ* 21 May, 296 6634:1419–20.

Cohen, I.B. (1948) *Science, Servant of Man*, Boston: Little Brown & Co.

Cole, G., Boyd, S., Kendall, B., Dinwiddie, R. and Matthews, D. (1984) Letter, *BMJ*, Dec. 8: 289.

Conference of Medical Royal Colleges and Their Faculties (1976) 'Diagnosis of brain death', *BMJ* 1:320.

Conference of Medical Royal Colleges and Their Faculties (1979) 'Diagnosis of death', *BMJ* 1:332.

Conference of Royal Medical Colleges and Their Faculties in the UK (1988) London: Department of Health and Social Security, *Report of a Working Party on Organ Transplantation in Neonates*.

Cranford, Ronald E., and Smith, Harmon L. (1979) 'Some critical distinctions between brain death and the persistent vegetative state', *Ethics in Science and Medicine* 6:199–209.

Dalyell, Tam, MP (1974) *Hansard*, Dec. 11.

Daws, Gavan (1983) ' "Animal liberation" as crime: the Hawaii dolphin case', in Harlan B. Miller and William H. Williams (eds) *Ethics and Animals*, New Jersey: Humana Press, 361–71.

Dougherty, John Jr., Rawlinson, G., Levy, David E., and Plum, Fred (1981) 'Hypoxic–ischemic brain injury and the vegetative state: clinical and neuropathologic correlation', *Neurology* 31, August:991–7.

Duckworth, Sir Dyce (1898) 'Some cases of cerebral disease in which the function of respiration entirely ceases for some hours before that of the circulation', *Edinburgh Medical Journal* 3:145–52.

Editorial (1968) 'After 25 centuries 1968 became the year of transplants', *Journal of the American Medical Association* 206 13, Dec. 23–30:2835.

The Ethics and Social Impact Committee Transplant Policy Center, Ann Arbor, MI (1988) 'Anencephalic infants as sources of transplantable organs', *Hastings Center Report* Oct./Nov.: 28–30.

Evans, Martyn (1989) 'Organ donation should not be restricted to relatives' *Journal of Medical Ethics* 15:17–20.

Feinberg, Joel (1985) 'The mistreatment of dead bodies', *Hastings Center Report* Feb.:31–7.

Fenigsen, Richard (1989) 'A case against Dutch euthanasia', *Hastings Center Report* Jan./Feb.:22–30.

Ferry, Georgina (1989) 'Brain grafters puzzled by their success', *New Scientist* 26 August:29.

Fine, Alan (1988) 'The ethics of fetal tissue transplants' *Hastings Center Report* June/July:5–8.

Fost, Norman (1988) 'Organs from anencephalic infants: an idea whose time has not yet come', *Hastings Center Report* Oct./Nov.:5–10.

Franklin, Cory (1988) 'Commentary', *Hastings Center Report* December:35–6.

Freund, Paul A. (1971) 'Organ transplants: ethical and legal problems', in Gorowtiz, Samuel, Macklin, Ruth, Jamton, Andrew L., O'Connor, John M., and Sherwin, Susan (eds) *Moral Problems in Medicine*, New Jersey: Prentice Hall.

Gervais, Karen G. (1987) *Redefining Death*, New Haven: Yale University Press.

Gil, Gideon (1989) 'The artificial heart juggernaut', *Hastings Center Report* March/April:24–31.

Gillett, G.R. (1986) 'Why let people die?', *Journal of Medical Ethics* 12:83–6.

Green, Michael B., and Wikler, Daniel (1981) 'Brain death and personal identity', in Cohen, Marshall, Nagel, Thomas and Scanlon, Thomas (eds) *Medicine and Moral Philosophy*, New Jersey: Princeton University Press, 49–77.

Hardy, James D., Chavez, Carlos M., Neely, William A., Erasian, Sadan, Turner, M. Don, Fabian, Leonard W., Labecki, Thaddeus D. (1964) 'Heart transplantation in man', *Journal of the American Medical Association*, 1132–39.

Harris, John (1985) *The Value of Life*, London: Routledge.

Harrison, Michael R. (1986) 'The anencephalic newborn as organ donor', *Hastings Center Report* April:21–2.

Jennett, B., Plum, F. (1972) 'The persistent vegetative state: a syndrome in search of a name', *Lancet* 1:734–7.

Jennett, Bryan (1987) Review of *Redefining Death*, *New Scientist* 2 July:62.

Jonas, Hans (1974) *Philosophical Essays: From Ancient Creed to Technological Man*, Englewood Cliffs, N.J.: Prentice Hall.

Jonsen, Albert R. (1988) 'Ethical issues in organ transplantation', in Veatch, Robert M. (ed.) *Medical Ethics*, Boston: Jones & Bartlett, 229–52.

Jouvet, M. (1959) 'Diagnostic electro-souscortico graphique de la mort du système nerveux-centrale aux cours de certains comas', *Electroencephalography and Clinical Neurophysiology* 11:805–8.

Kass, Leon R. (1985) 'Thinking about the body', *Hastings Center Report*, Feb.: 20–30.

Kennedy, Ian (1988) *Treat Me Right: Essays in Medical Law and Ethics*, Oxford: Clarendon.

King, Nancy P.P. (1987) 'Federal and State regulations of neonatal decision-making', in McMillan, R.C., Engelhardt Jr., H.T. and Spicker, S.F. (eds) *Euthanasia and the Newborn*, Doordrecht: Reidel, 89–115.

Kirkpatrick, Charles H. (1987) 'Transplantation immunology', *Journal of the American Medical Association* Nov. 27, 258 20:2993–3000.

Koop, C. Everett (1982) Statements Before the Hearing on Handicapped Newborns, Subcommittee on Select Education Committee and Labor, US House of Representatives, September 16.

Korein, J. (1978) 'The problems of brain death', *Annals of the New York Academy of Sciences* 315:19–38.

Kuhse, H., and Singer, P. (1985) *Should the Baby Live?*, Oxford: OUP.

Kushner, T. (1984) 'Having a life versus being alive', *Journal of Medical Ethics* 10:5–8.

Kushner, Thomasine, and Belliotti, Raymond (1985) 'Baby Fae: a beastly business', *Journal of Medical Ethics* 11:178–83.

Lamb, D. (1978) 'Diagnosing death', *Philosophy and Public Affairs*, Winter, 7 2:144–53.

——(1985) *Death, Brain Death and Ethics*, London: Croom Helm.

——(1988) *Down the Slippery Slope*, London: Croom Helm.

Lamb, D., and Easton, S.M. (1984) *Multiple Discovery: The Pattern of Scientific Progress*, Aldershot: Gower/Avebury.

Landwirth, Julius (1988) 'Should anencephalic infants be used as organ donors?', *Pediatrics* August 82 2:257–9.

Lemire, Ronald J., Beckwith, J. Bruce, and Warkany, Joseph (1978) *Anencephaly*, New York: Raven Press.

Levy, D.E., Carronna, J.J., and Singer, B.H. (1985) 'Predicting outcome from hypoxic–ischemic coma', *Journal of the American Medical Association* 253:1420–6.

Levy, David E., Sidtis, John J., Rottenberg, A., Jarden, Jens D., Strother, Stephen C., Dhawen, Vijay, Ginos, James Z., Tramo, Mark J., Evans, Alan C., and Plum, Fred (1987) 'Differences in cerebral blood flow and glucose utilization in vegetative versus locked-in patients', *Annals of Neurology* 22 6, December:673–82.

Lynn, J. (1983) 'The determination of death', *Annals of Internal Medicine*, 99 2:264–6.

Lyons, Catherine (1970) *Organ Transplants: The Moral Issues*, London: SCM Press.

McCormick, R. (1974) 'To save or let die?: the dilemma of modern medicine', *Journal of the American Medical Association* 229:172–6.

McLennan Report (1969) *Advice on the Question of Amending The Human Tissue Act 1961*, CMMD 4106, London: HMSO.

Milunsky, Aubrey (1988) 'Harvesting organs from dying anencephalic infants', *Pediatrics* August 82 12:274–6.

Mohandas, A., and Chou, S.N. (1971) *Journal of Neurosurgery* 35:211–18.

Mollaret, P., and Goulon, M. (1959) 'Le coma dépassé', *Revue Neurologique*, 101:3–15.

Moore, Francis D., et al. (1968) 'Cardiac and other organ transplantation', *Journal of the American Medical Association* 206 11, Dec. 9:2489–90.

Morison, R.S. (1971) 'Death: process or event?', *Science* 173:694–8.

Moulavi, M.H., Babu Sahib (1984) 'Organ donation: an Islamic viewpoint', Newsletter of the *National Kidney Foundation*, Singapore, 1 2:1–5.

The National Commission For The Protection of Human Subjects of Biomedical and Behavioural Research (1975) *Research on the Fetus: Appendix*, US Department of Health, Education and Welfare Publication (OS) 76–128, Government Printing Office.

New York State Task Force on Life and the Law (1988) *Transplantation in New York State: The Procurement and Distribution of Organs and Tissues*, New York, Jan.

Nolan, Kathleen (1988) 'Genug is genug: a fetus is not a kidney', *Hastings Center Report* December:13–19.

Pallis, C. (1980) quoted in 'News and Notes', *BMJ* 282:1220.

____(1983) *The ABC of Brainstem Death*, London: BMJ.

____(1984) 'Brainstem death: the evolution of a concept', in Morris, Peter J. (ed.) *Kidney Transplantation: Principles and Practice*, 2nd edition, London: Grune and Stratton, 101–27.

____(1985) 'Defining Death', *BMJ* 291:666–7.

____(1987) Entry on 'Death' in *Encyclopaedia Britannica*, Chicago, 1030–42.

____(1989) Personal communication.

Pallis, C., and Prior, P.F. (1983) 'Guidelines for the determination of death: an appraisal', *Neurology* 33:251.

Polkinghorne, John (1988) *Review of the Guidance on the Research Use of Foetuses and Foetal Matter*, London: HMSO.

Pope Pius XII (1958) 'The prolongation of life', An Address of Pope Pius XII to an International Congress of Anaesthesiologists, *The Pope Speaks*, 4 November 1957:393–8.

Posner, Jerome B. (1978) 'Coma and other states of consciousness: the differential diagnosis of brain death', *New York Academy of Sciences* 315:215–27.

President's Commission For The Study of Ethical Problems on Medicine and Biomedical and Behavioural Research (1981) *Defining Death*, Washington, and (1983) *Decisions to Forego Life-sustaining Therapy*.

Puccetti, R. (1976) 'The conquest of death', *Monist* 59 2:249–63.

____(1988) 'Neo-cortical death' in Zaner, Richard M. (ed.) *Death: Beyond Whole Brain Criteria*, Dordrecht: Kluwer, 75–90.

Rachels, James (1986) *The End of Life*, Oxford: OUP.

Ramsey, Paul (1970) *The Patient as Person*, New Haven: Yale University Press.

Report from the King's Fund Panel (1989), *Intensive Care in the United Kingdom*, May, London: King's Fund Centre.

Report of the Conference of European Health Ministers, Council of Europe (1987) 'Ethical and Socio-Cultural Problems Raised by Organ Transplantation', Paris, 16–17 November.

Report of the Swedish Committee on Defining Death (1984) *The Concept of Death Summary*, The Swedish Ministry of Health and Social Affairs.

Robertson, John A. (1988) 'Rights, symbolism and public policy in fetal tissue transplants', *Hastings Center Report* December:5–12.

Rolston, H. (1982) 'The irreversible comatose: respect for the subhuman in human life', *Journal of Medical Philosophy* 7:337.

Rosenberg, G.A., Johnson, S.F., and Brenner, R.P. (1977) 'Recovery of cognition after prolonged vegetative state', *Annals of Neurology* 2:167–8.

Salaman, J.R. (1989) 'Anencephalic organ donors: guidelines available from Britain and North America', *BMJ* 298 11 March: 622–3.

Sandler, B. (1968) 'Cardiac transplantation', *Lancet* 551:1086–7.

Schroeder, John Speer, and Hunt, Sharon (1987) 'Cardiac transplantation', *Journal of the American Medical Association* Dec.4 258 21:3142–5.

Schwartz, H.S. (1985) 'Bioethical and legal considerations in increasing the supply of transplantable organs: from UAGA to baby Fae', *American Journal of Law and Medicine* 10:397–438.

Sells, R. (1979) 'Let's not opt out: kidney donation and transplantation', *Journal of Medical Ethics* 5 2:165–9.

Shaw, Margery, W. (1987) 'When does treatment constitute a harm?', in McMillan, Richard C. *et al.*, *Euthanasia and the Newborn*, Dordrecht: D. Reidel, 117–37.

Shewmon, Alan D. (1988) 'Anencephaly: selected medical aspects', *Hastings Center Report* Oct./Nov.:11–18.

Shewmon, Alan D., Capron, Alexander M., Peacock, Wawrick J., Schulman, Barbara L. (1989) 'The use of anencephalic infants as organ sources', *Journal of the American Medical Association* 261, 12: 1173–81.

Skipworth, Mark (1989) 'Suicide on prescription', *Observer Magazine* 30 April:18–22.

Smith, David Randolph (1988) 'Legal issues leading to the notion of neocortical death', in Zaner, Richard M. (ed.) *Death: Beyond Whole Brain Criteria*, Dordrecht: Kluwer, 111–44.

Stanley, John M. (1987) 'More fiddling with the definition of death?', *Journal of Medical Ethics* 13:21–2.

Starzl, Thomas E. (1985) 'Will living organ donations no longer be justified?', *Hastings Center Report* April:5.

Task Force on Death and Dying of the Institute of Society, Ethics and The Life Sciences (1977) 'Refinements in criteria for the determination of death: an appraisal', in Weir, R.F. (ed.) *Ethical Issues in Death and Dying*, New York: Columbia University Press, 80–102.

Taussig, Helen B. (1969) 'A time for waiting', *The Johns Hopkins Magazine* Spring:9–11.

Titmus, Richard M. (1971) *The Gift Relationship*, London: Allen & Unwin.

Toledo-Pereyra, Luis (ed.) (1987) *Complications of Organ Transplantation* (Immunology Series, 32) New York: Dekker.

Tooley, Michael (1973) 'A defence of abortion and infanticide' in Feinberg, J. (ed.) *The Problem of Abortion*, Belmont CA.: Wadsworth Publishing Co., 51–91.

Varga, Andrew C. (1984) *The Main Issues in Bioethics*, revised edition, New York: Paulist Press.

Veatch, R.M. (1976) *Death, Dying and the Biological Revolution*, New Haven and London: Yale University Press.

——(1978) 'The definition of death: ethical and philosophical and policy confusion', *Annals of the New York Academy of Sciences* 315:307–21.

Vincenti, Flavio, Parfrey, Patrick, and Briggs, William (1986) 'Skeletal gastrointestinal, hepatic and hematologic disorders following kidney transplantation', in Garovoy, Martin, and Guttmann, Ronald (eds) *Renal Transplantation*, New York: Churchill Livingstone, 233–71.

Walker, A. Earl (1979) 'Advances in the determination of death', in

Thompson, R.A. and Green, J.R. (eds) *Advances in Neurology* 22, New York: Raven Press, 167–77.

Walker, A. Earl, Feeny, Dennis M., and Hovda, David A. (1984) 'The electroencephalographic characteristics of the rhombencephalectomized cat', *Electroencephalography and Clinical Neurophysiology* 57:158–65.

Walters, James W. and Ashwal, Stephen (1988) 'Organ prolongation in anencephalic infants: ethical and medical issues', *Hastings Center Report* Oct./Nov.:19–27.

Walton, D.N. (1980) *Brain Death*, Indiana: Purdue University Press.

Warkany, Josef (1971) *Congenital Malformations*, Chicago: Year Book Medical Publishers.

Weiss, Ann E. (1985) *Bioethics: Dilemmas in Modern Medicine*, NJ.: Enslow Publishers, inc.

Wertheimer, P., Jouvet, M., and Descotes, J. (1959) 'A propos du diagnostic de la mort du système nerveux', *Presse Médicale* 67:87–8.

White, Robert J. (1983) 'Individualità e trapianto cerebrale', *Trapianto di Cuore e Trapianto di Cervello*, Orizzonte Medico: Vatican, 102–130.

Willke, J.C., and Andrusko, Dave (1988) 'Personhood redux', *Hastings Center Report* October/November:30–3.

Woodhouse, Mark B. (1987) 'Philosophy and frontier science: is there a new paradigm in the making?', *Explorations in Knowledge* IV 2:1–18.

Yanchinski, Stephanie (1988) 'Fetal tissue may not be needed for Parkinson's', *New Scientist* 3 December:32.

Younger, S.J., and Bartlett, E.T. (1983) 'Human death and high technology: the failure of the whole brain formulations, *Annals of Internal Medicine* 99:252–8.

Zaner, R.M. (ed.) (1988) *Death: Beyond Whole Brain Criteria*, Dordrecht: Kluwer, 111–44.

SUBJECT INDEX

NAME INDEX

Anderson, I. 17, 152
Andrusko, D. 95, 99, 158
Angelini, Monsignor 104
Annas, G. 86, 91, 93, 146–7, 152
Aristotle 3
Arnold, J. D. 31, 152
Ashwal, S. 86, 89, 158

Barnard, C. 12, 22
Beckwith, J. 97, 155
Belliotti, R. 112, 155
Bentham, J. 3
Beresford, H. R. 53, 152
Blaiberg, P. 12
Botkin, J. R. 83–4, 95, 101, 152
Bradley, B. A. 11, 149, 152
Briggs, W. 12, 157
Browne, A. 32, 38, 152

Calne, Sir Roy 16–17, 152
Caplan, A. L. 91, 127, 153
Capron, A. M. 82, 90–1, 93, 98–9, 119–20, 153
Carrel, A. 8
Carse, J. P. 28, 153
Chisholm, G. B. 127, 140, 153
Chou, S. N. 34, 155
Clarke, B. 20–1, 115–16
Cohen, I. B. 112, 153
Cole, G. B. 56, 153
Cushing, H. 32

Dalyell, T. 143–4, 153
Dark, J. 14–15, 112, 127–8
Daws, G. 49, 153
Denys, J. B. 111–12

Dougherty, J. 54–5, 153
Duckworth, Sir Dyce 32, 153

Easton, S. M. 111, 155
Evans, M. 110, 153

Fae, Baby 112
Feinberg, J. 123–4, 153
Fenigsen, R. 5, 153
Ferry, G. 72, 153
Fine, A. 70, 72–3, 76, 154
Fost, N. 85, 88, 94, 154
Franklin, C. 15, 132, 154
Freund, P.A. 130, 154

Gabriel, Baby 82–3
Gervais, K. G. 44–6, 57–9, 65, 92, 154
Gil, G. O. 115, 154
Gillett, G. R. 61, 63–4, 154
Goodman, E. 82
Goulon, M. 32, 155
Gove, A. 134
Green, M. B. 46, 154
Guthrie, C. 8

Hardy, J. D. 112, 154
Harris, J. 78–9, 154
Harrison, M. J. 93, 154
Herrick, R. 10
Hume, D. 10
Hunt, S. 15–16, 148, 157

Jacobs, H. B. 134
James, W. 124
Jennett, B. 38, 154

161